Fitness Sutra

STRENGTH TRAINING WITH DUMBBELLS

50+ Exercises to Build Muscle, Burn Fat
& Sculpt your Body at Home

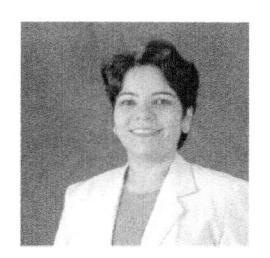

Dr. Monika Chopra
www.fitness-sutra.com

Dr. Monika Chopra's Fitness Sutra

Copyright © Dr. Monika Chopra, 2019. All rights reserved.

Published by FitSutra Wellness Pvt Ltd,
33, Prachi Residency, Baner Rd., Pune-411045, India

ISBN-13: 978-1-0956-6477-3

No part of this book may be reproduced, transmitted, or utilized in any form or by any means, electronic or mechanical including photocopying or recording or by any information storage and retrieval system, without written permission from the author.

Although I am a Physiotherapist (PT, for those of you in the USA) and a trained Yoga teacher, my suggestions through this book do not establish a doctor-patient relationship between us. This book is not intended to be a substitute for the medical advice of physicians. You should regularly consult a physician in matters relating to your health particularly with respect to any symptoms that may require diagnosis or medical attention. I advise you to take full responsibility of your safety and be aware of your physical limits. Before practising the exercises described in this book, be sure that your equipment is well maintained. Do not take risks beyond your level of flexibility, aptitude, strength, and comfort level.

This is a work of nonfiction. No names have been changed, no characters invented and no events fabricated. The information provided within this Book is for general informational purposes only. While I have tried to keep the information up-to-date and correct, there are no representations or warranties, expressed or implied, about the completeness, accuracy, reliability, suitability or availability with respect to the information, products, services, or related graphics contained in this book for any purpose. Any use of this information is at the reader's own responsibility. I do not assume and hereby disclaim any liability to any party for any loss, damage, or disruption caused by errors or omissions, whether such errors or omissions result from negligence, accident, or any other cause.

Strength Training with Dumbbells

CONTENTS

1	Introduction to Strength Training	1
2	Why Exercise with Dumbbells	6
3	Warm-Up Exercises	11
4	Upper Body Exercises	21
	Hammer-Curl	22
	Split Stance Dumbbell Curl	24
	Reverse Biceps Curl	26
	Seated Dumbbell Triceps Extension	28
	Bent-over Triceps Kickback	30
	Seated Side Lateral Raise	32
	Alternate Dumbbell Incline Bench Press	34
	Dumbbell L-Arm Lateral Raise	36
	Overhead Dumbbell Press	38
	Seated Overhead Dumbbell Press	40
	Side Lying Lateral Raise	42
	Dumbbell Pull Over the Head	44
	Upright Row	46
	Dumbbell Swing	48
	Dumbbell Front Raise	50
	Dumbbell Shoulder Shrug	52
	Seated Dumbbell Palm-up Wrist Curl	54
	Dumbbell Bench Press	56
	Flat Dumbbell Crush Press	58
	Incline Dumbbell Chest Fly	60
	Dumbbell "T" Push-Ups	62
	Dumbbell Rowing	64
	Renegade Row	66
	Supported Incline Chest Dumbbell Row	68

	3-point Support Dumbbell Row	70
	Bent-over Dumbbell Sideways Raise	72
5	Lower Body Exercises	75
	Dumbbell Diagonal Lunge	76
	Walking Dumbbell Lunge	78
	Dumbbell Lunge and Rotation	80
	Dumbbell Step	82
	Side Lunge Jump off	84
	Goblet Squat with Pulses	86
	Curtsy Lunge	88
	Bulgarian Split Lunge	90
	Romanian Deadlift	92
	Single Leg Dumbbell Deadlift	94
	Weighted Bridge Lift	96
	Standing Dumbbell Calf Raise	98
6	Core Exercises	101
	Dumbbell Side Plank Reach Rotate	102
	Negative Sit-up	104
	Dumbbell Sit-ups	106
	Sit-ups with Dumbbells	108
7	Full Body Exercises	111
	Dumbbell Raise with Jump	112
	Dumbbell One Arm Raise	114
	Half Turkish Get-up Dumbbell Raise	116
	Dumbbell Chop	118
	Single Arm Dumbbell Snatch	120
	Overhead Dumbbell Squat	122
	Dumbbell Split Jump	124
	Dumbbell Reverse Lunge High Knee & Press	126
	Dumbbell Full Squat Press	128

		Jumping Jacks with Dumbbells	130
		Dumbbell Windmill	132
	8	Cool-Down Exercises	134
	9	Importance of Diet	142
	10	Training Regimes	145
	11	Bonus	152

Dr. Monika Chopra's Fitness Sutra

CHAPTER 1

Introduction to Strength Training

Dr. Monika Chopra's Fitness Sutra

Importance of Strength Training

1. Strength training helps to reverse the loss of muscle mass which decreases with age naturally.

2. Increased muscle strength improves your posture with upright spine & helps in attaining that "V" shaped body.

3. A muscular, leaner & fitter body helps in your notion of "Self-Image" and leads to higher self-esteem & confidence.

4. Strength training helps to increase bone density thereby reducing the risk of osteoporosis & fractures.

5. Strength training helps to maintain joint flexibility and can reduce the symptoms of arthritis.

6. As you gain muscle, your base metabolic rate tends to increase, thus making it easier to control your weight. This single factor can prevent a lot of potential issues related to obesity & being overweight - first & foremost of which is Diabetes.

7. Strength training when paired with cardiovascular training helps in strengthening alternative arterial passages in your heart thereby reducing blood pressure and risk of blocked arteries.

Strength Training with Dumbbells

8. Strength training can help alleviate chronic pains like low back pain & joint pains.

9. Strength training helps in reversal in mitochondrial deterioration that typically occurs with aging.

10. Strength training improves the movement of lymphatic fluid through your system thus aiding in efficient removal of toxins.

11. Strength training releases endorphins in brain. Endorphins act as our natural defences towards stress and depression. Endorphins are the reason why you feel happy & satisfied after a productive session of strength training.

12. Strength training reduces oxidative stress thus reducing risks of cancer.

13. Strength training helps you to get good night sleep thus having overall positive impact on your health.

Safety Tips for Strength Training

1. <u>Warm up routine</u> is very important before any strength training regime. It helps to increase blood flow to joints and muscles, prepares joints for performance by improving joint mobility, activates your core and hip muscles to provide better stability to spine and hips.

2. <u>Using proper form</u> during strength training is very important to minimize injuries and maximize gains. The exercises should be practised with lower resistance first to master the form for that routine and then only should you move to increased resistance.

3. <u>Working at right tempo</u> helps to maximize the strength gains with momentum not interfering with the motive of exercise. Always count slowly as you perform the exercise, thus controlling movement and give a slight pause in between as you reach at maximum resistance effect. Do not let the momentum of the movement carry on till the end. Never lose control of the movement.

4. <u>Keep breathing</u> slowly and never hold your breath during exercise to avoid build-up of your blood pressure. Generally, you should exhale as you work against resistance & inhale as you release.

5. Keep challenging the muscles by <u>slowly increasing the resistance</u>. The choice of resistance should be such that at the end of one set of repetition the targeted muscle or group of muscles should be tired (but not too tired) and the exercise can still be performed in proper form. When you feel the resistance becoming easier, add more resistance or add a set.

Strength Training with Dumbbells

6. Ideally you should <u>workout all major muscle groups</u> of your body 2-3 times a week. This can be done by dividing regimes into upper and lower body muscles components and doing them on separate days, repeating each component at least 2-3 times a week or doing full body exercises 2-3 times a week.

7. Tiny tears occur in muscle tissues due to strength training which need to be healed. These tears make the muscles grow stronger after re-modelling. At least 48 hours should be given to each muscle to recover before further strength training.

8. <u>Cut back</u> on the exercise (reduce resistance or reduce the sets) if you feel significant pain, dizziness, breathlessness during the session or feel tired throughout the day.

9. Always keep a <u>slight bend in knees and elbows</u> while straightening arms and legs during exercises. Locking these joints at the extreme ends of your resistance exercise can lead to injuries.

10. <u>Cool down</u> with full body stretches after the session. 5-10 minutes cool down exercises should be good.

CHAPTER 2

Why Exercise with Dumbbells

Strength Training with Dumbbells

Dumbbell exercise program is an effective, convenient, and an inexpensive way of doing the strength training workout. You do not necessarily need an elaborate gym setup to do the exercises. It can easily be done at home or your workplace.

In this book, through step by step instructions, I will guide you to the safe and effective methods of using Dumbbells for Strength Training. Emphasis will be laid on the correct grasping of the dumbbell, proper start position and correct movement of the particular body part for the desired results.

Finally I will guide you to beginners, intermediate and advance training regimes which will help you to set desired goals.

Why to Choose the Correct Dumbbell Weight:

Choosing the correct dumbbell weight is very important to get the desired results from the exercises. Less dumbbell weight may lead to ineffective outcomes towards muscle strengthening, endurance etc. On the other side a very heavy dumbbell can lead to muscle strains and joint injuries.

How to Choose a Correct Dumbbell Weight:

To understand how to choose the dumbbell weight we first need to understand how exercises are performed. Dumbbell exercises are done as sets of repetitions. A repetition is completing one exercise and a set is a group of repetitions.

The choice of a particular dumbbell weight depends on how comfortably you can complete a set of 8-10 repetitions with the chosen weight. With the correct weight you should be able to do 8-10 repetitions comfortably (but not too comfortably also). At the end of the set your muscles start feeling tired and you may struggle a bit to complete the set.

You can make out if the dumbbell is too heavy when you start straining your back or swinging your body to lift the weight or perform the exercise.

Important Tips for Dumbbell Exercise Program

- Complete the regime at least twice a week to get appropriate results. Any number less than that may not be beneficial and you may feel demotivated to continue.

- Once you are comfortable with the exercises (that is, you have built up enough stamina and strength), repeat the sessions 3-4 times a week.

- Be prepared to feel little sore in muscles and also sometimes joints as you start with the exercise program. This is normal and may subside in a day or two. As you continue with the sessions the exercises will become easier and more comfortable.

Strength Training with Dumbbells

- Rest for a day between the sessions. Once you've built up the stamina and strength you may do 3-4 sessions a week.

- Try switching dumbbell workout with cardiovascular training. Going for walks on alternate days with dumbbell workout helps to build your stamina. Even with this, take 1-2 days of rest in a week. Do not overstrain.

- Reduce number of sets but perform all the exercises if you feel too much strained with the regime. In case of any medical reason to stop a particular exercise, replace the exercise with some other exercise.

- Ensure proper hydration. Do not let yourself get dehydrated during exercise. Replenish any loss of water through sweat with water or electrolytes.

- Wear appropriate footwear while exercising especially if you are diabetic, have flat foot or have pronated foot.

Bonus

I hope you are finding this book useful and are ready to start with the exercises.

I have also created easy to use quick reference charts of the regimes (beginners / intermediate / advanced), suggested in the last chapter of this book. These can be downloaded as ready printable files from

https://www.fitness-sutra.com/go?id=131064

SCAN ME!

You can also subscribe to my mailing list to get more tips & motivation to do these exercises. I try to keep my subscribers abreast of the latest developments in the field of strength training.

CHAPTER 3

Warm-Up Exercises

To stay safe and prepare your body for exercises you should always do some warm ups before the strength exercises. The warm up exercises help to increase the temperature and loosen the muscles before the heavy body muscle work. Warm ups improve the body performance and prevent injuries. These exercises should be dynamic exercises like skipping, jogging at a place, chest expansion & rotations. About 5 minutes' warm ups are enough to make your cardiovascular system ready.

The following warm up exercises are good to prepare your body for an intense workout.

1. <u>Neck Rotations:</u>

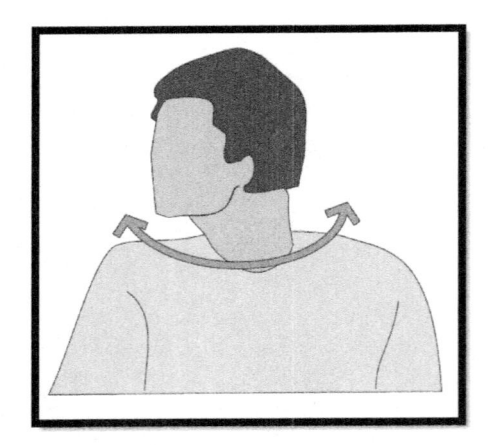

Stand tall with your chin parallel to the ground. Exhale and take your chin to the chest. Inhale, rotate your neck and take your chin towards the left shoulder (look over your left shoulder). Exhale and get your chin back to the chest position. Inhale, rotate your neck and take your chin to the right shoulder (look over your right shoulder). Get your chin back to the chest position as you exhale. Move you chin up to the start position as you inhale. Repeat 3 times.

Strength Training with Dumbbells

2. <u>Shoulder Backward Rotations:</u>

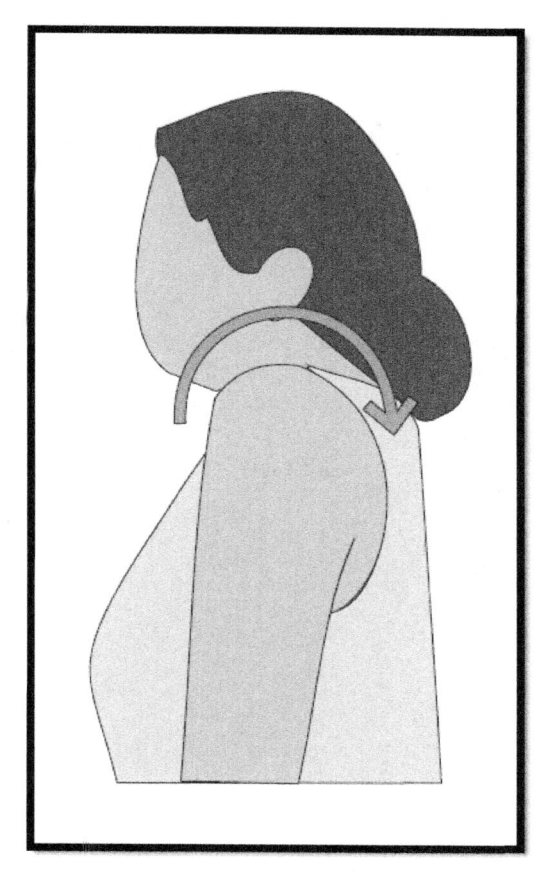

Stand tall with chin parallel to the floor and shoulders facing forward. Take your shoulders forward. Start rotating the shoulders taking them up and behind. Get your shoulder-blades together as you move the shoulders behind. Get shoulders back to the start position.

3. <u>Shoulder Forward Rotations:</u>

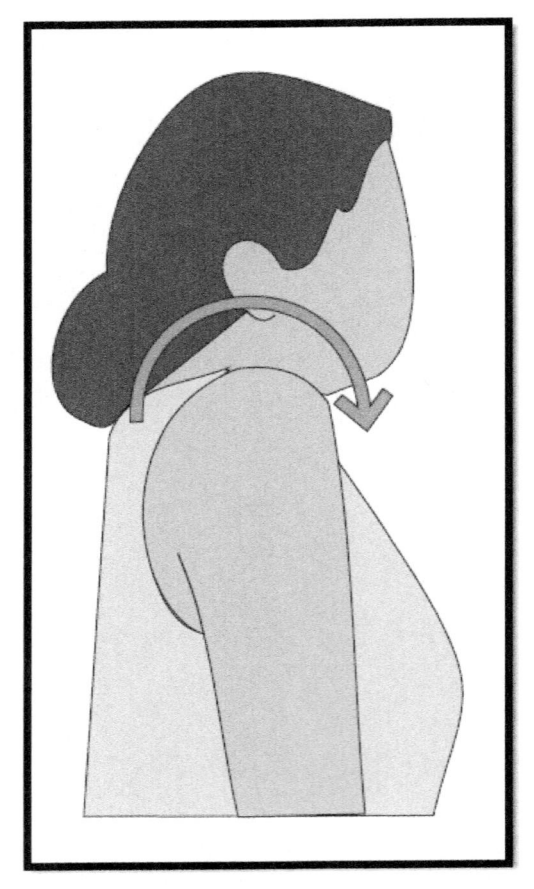

Stand tall with chin parallel to the floor and shoulders facing forward. Take your shoulders behind, getting your shoulder blades together. Continue rotating the shoulders taking them up and forwards. Get shoulders back to the start position. Repeat this sequence 10 times.

Strength Training with Dumbbells

4. <u>Chest Expansions:</u>

Stand tall with chin parallel to the floor and shoulders facing forward. Raise your arms to the shoulder level and take them back opening the chest. Repeat 10 times.

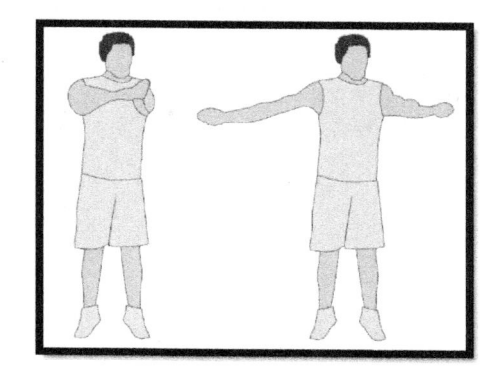

5. <u>Torso Rotations:</u>

Stand tall with feet hip width distance apart. Place your hands on the waist and rotate your trunk clockwise. Repeat 10 times. Then rotate your trunk anti-clockwise. Repeat 10 times.

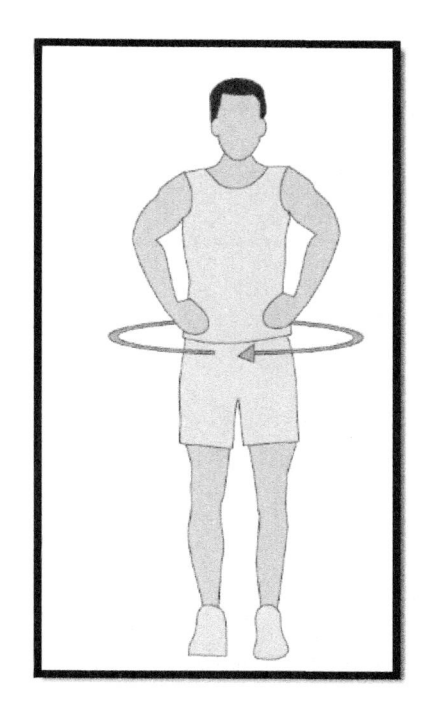

Dr. Monika Chopra's Fitness Sutra

6. <u>Arm Rotations:</u>

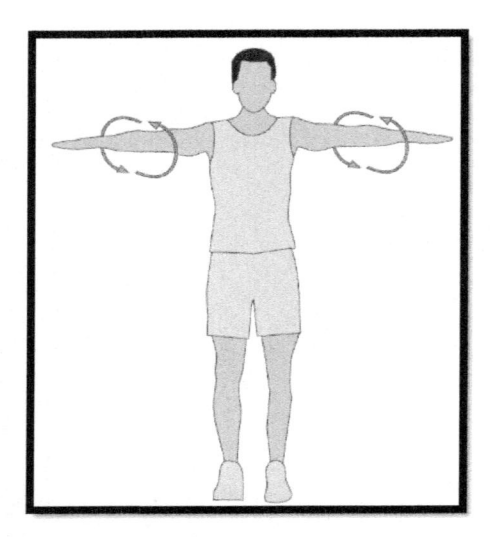

Stand tall with your feet hip width distance apart. Raise your arms to the side at shoulder level. Make circles with your arms moving them clockwise and anti-clockwise (10 times in each direction).

7. <u>Side Arm Raises:</u>

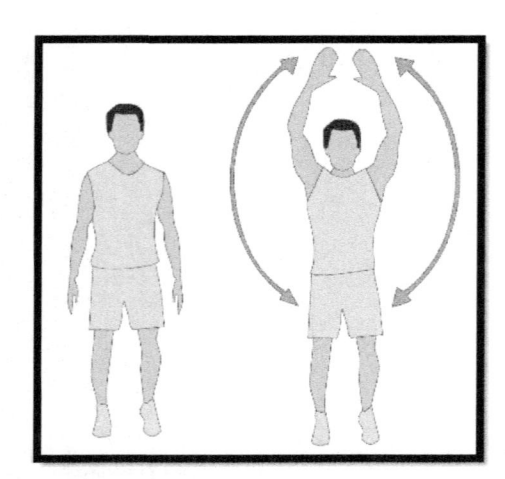

Stand tall with your feet hip width distance apart. Raise your both arms sideways up 10 times.

8. <u>Hip Rotation</u>

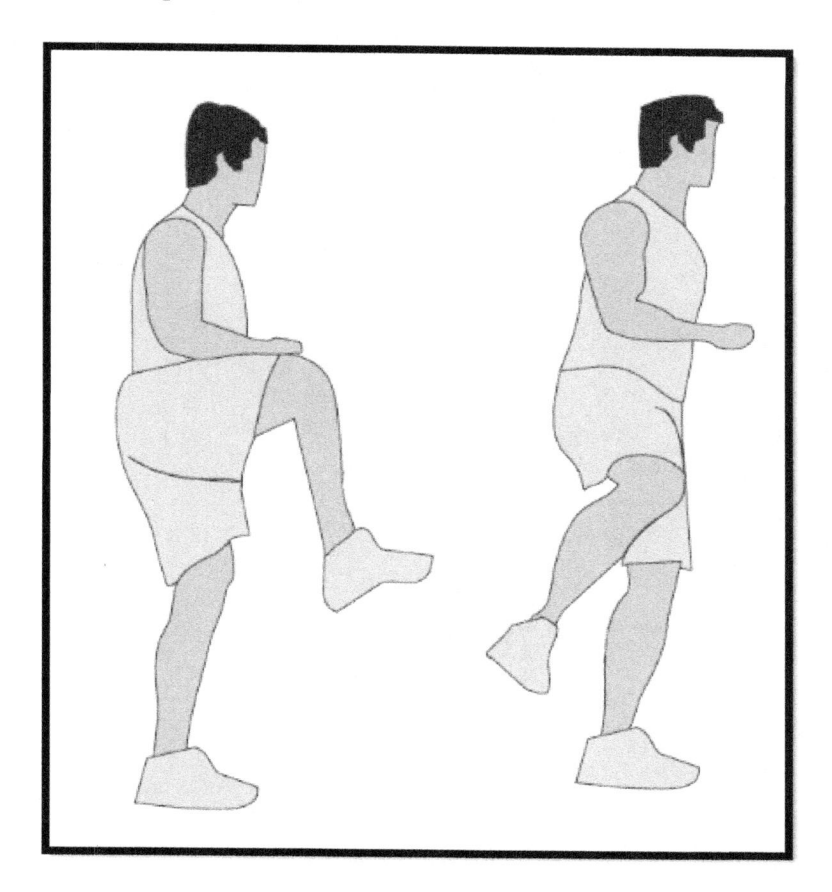

Lift your right leg and balance your body on the left foot. Rotate your leg at the hips in clockwise direction 10 times. Next rotate it in reverse direction 10 times. Repeat with the other leg.

9. Jog on Spot

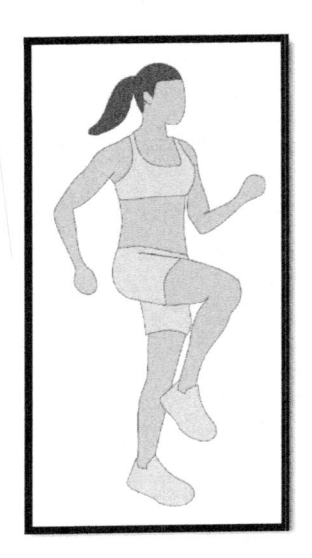

Jog on the spot. Try to lift your legs high enough to make your thighs parallel to the ground. Do 20 jogs of each foot.

10. Side to Side Hop

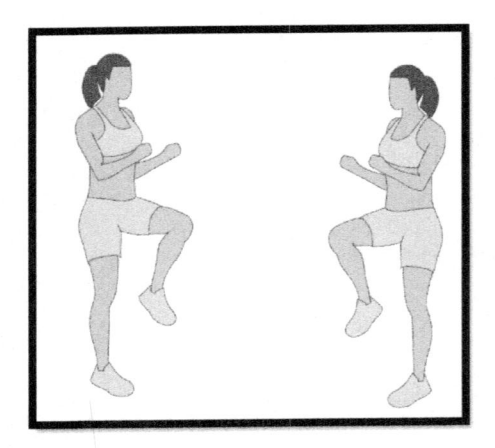

Balance yourself on one foot with the other leg raised high. Hop on the raised leg side, bringing that one down and raising the other leg up simultaneously. Repeat this 20 times.

Strength Training with Dumbbells

<u>Warm-up Sets</u>: Every exercise you want to perform should begin with a warm up set. Warm up set includes all the exercises you are going to do, with little or no resistance for 10-15 repetitions with slower than normal tempo.

Dr. Monika Chopra's Fitness Sutra

"I work out a lot, but it changes day to day. I always start out with some cardio - either a jog, a bike ride, or footwork drills designed specifically for tennis movement. Then I do weights, but I switch the days: one day it's upper body, the next day it's lower body. Then I do stomach and back pretty much every day."

- Ana Ivanovic

CHAPTER 4

Upper Body Exercises

Biceps & Forearm Exercises

Hammer-Curl

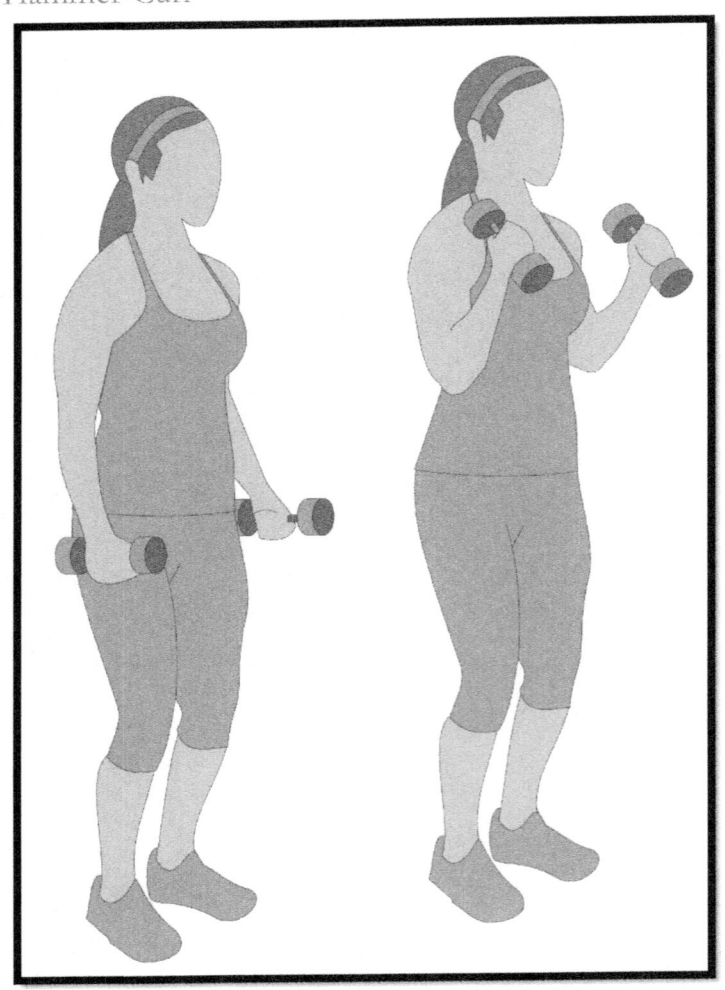

Strength Training with Dumbbells

Effect: Strengthening of biceps and forearm muscles.

Difficulty Level: Beginner

Start Position: Grab dumbbells in the neutral grip with palms facing inward, arms hanging by side of your body and stand tall with feet hip width distance apart.

Steps:

1. Brace your core and curl your arms at elbows with the elbows tucked by the sides of your body, taking the dumbbells to shoulder level.
2. Pause and feel the contraction in biceps.
3. Slowly uncurl the arms taking dumbbells down to the start position.

Fine Tips:

1. Keep the core braced and avoid bending backwards as you do the movement.
2. Keep your elbows tucked by the side of your body throughout the movement.
3. The movement should be slow and controlled avoiding momentum to contribute to the range.

Split Stance Dumbbell Curl

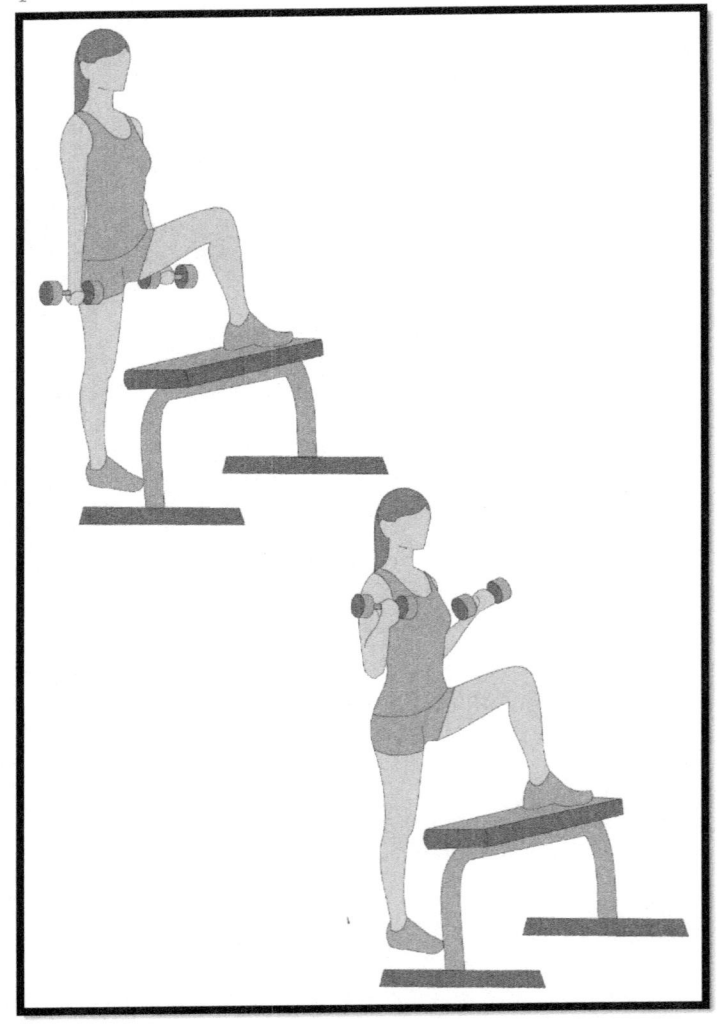

Strength Training with Dumbbells

Effect: Strengthening of biceps with increased stability of lower body.

Difficulty Level: Intermediate

Start Position: Grab a pair of dumbbells with palms facing forward & arms by the side of your body. Stand in a split stance with one foot on the bench, back tall and core engaged.

Steps:

1. Brace your core and curl your arms at the elbows taking the dumbbells to the shoulder keeping the arms tucked by the side of the body.
2. Return to the start position.
3. Repeat required number of times and switch the legs.

Fine Tips:

1. Keep your back tall and abdomen tucked in throughout the exercise.
2. Keep the elbows tucked by the side of your body during movement.
3. The movement should be slow and controlled.

Dr. Monika Chopra's Fitness Sutra

Reverse Biceps Curl

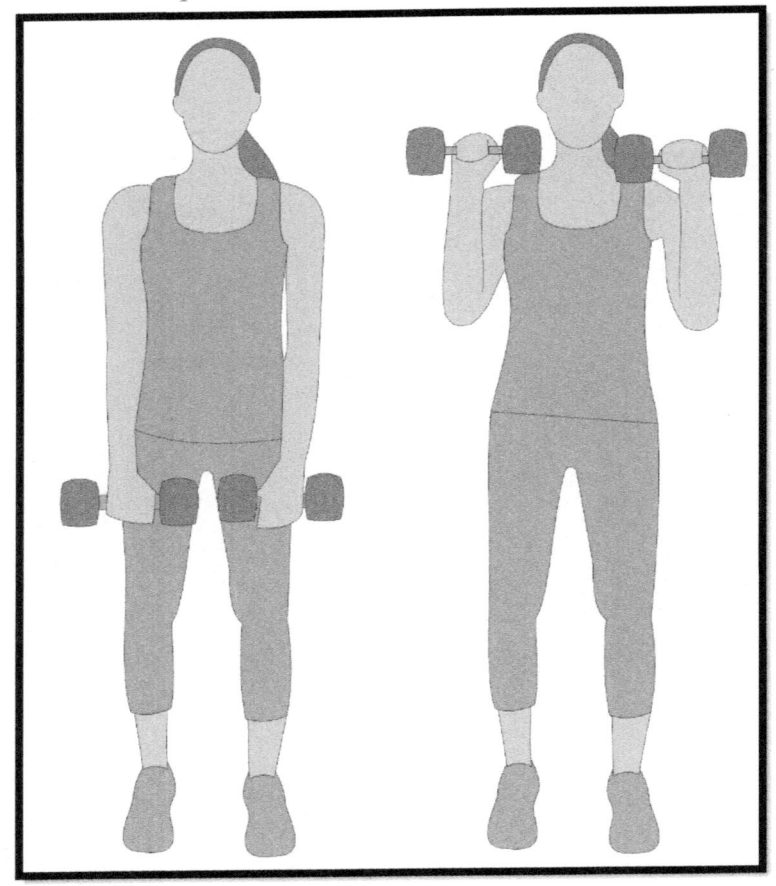

Strength Training with Dumbbells

Effect: This exercise focuses on strengthening biceps, brachialis and brachioradialis muscles.

Difficulty Level: Beginner

Start Position: Grab dumbbells in your hands, shoulder width apart with palms facing down (pronated grip) and arms extended with the elbows by the side of your body.

Steps:

1. Keeping the upper arms stationary, curl the dumbbells up by contracting the biceps till the dumbbells reach the shoulder level.
2. Pause in the top position.
3. Slowly reverse the movement and come to the start position.
4. Repeat required number of times.

Fine Tips:

1. The movement should be slow and controlled with momentum not aiding in the movement.
2. Keep your elbows tucked by the side of the body and upper arms stationary as you do the movement.

Triceps & Forearm Exercises

Seated Dumbbell Triceps Extension

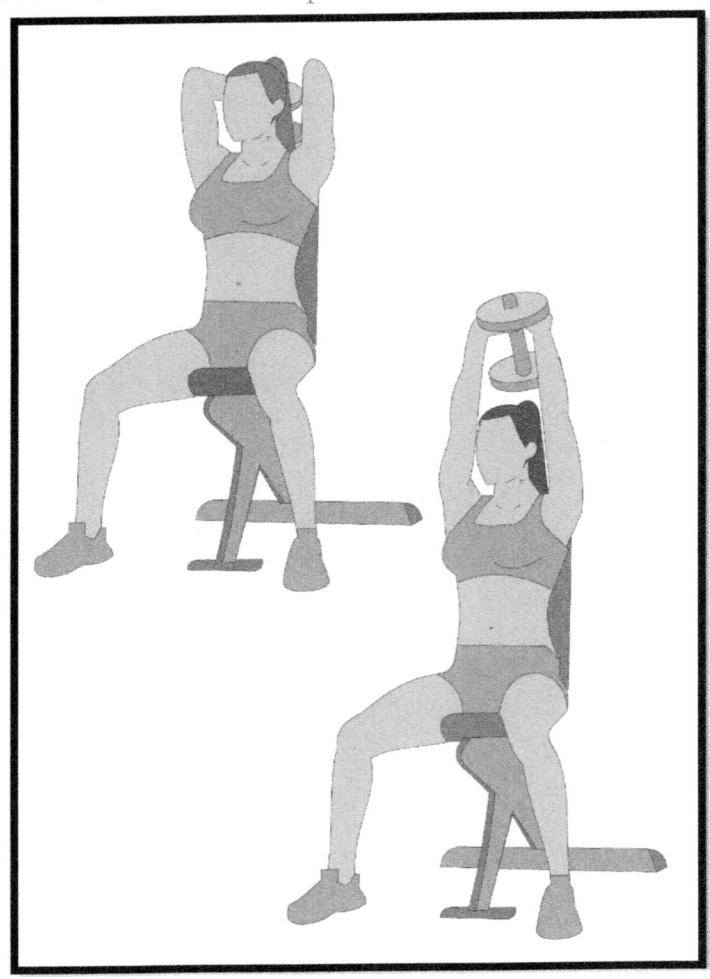

Strength Training with Dumbbells

Effect: This exercise focuses on strengthening of triceps muscles along with improving the stability and mobility of shoulder.

Difficulty Level: Beginner

Start Position: Grab a dumbbell in your hands overhead and sit tall on the bench with back supported.

Steps:

1. Raise the dumbbell straightening your arms overhead.
2. Pause in the highest position.
3. Bend the arms at elbow and lower the dumbbell till behind the neck.
4. Repeat required number of times.

Fine Tips:

1. The movement should be slow and steady without momentum helping in the movement.
2. Keep the upper arms steady as you lower the dumbbell behind your neck.
3. Feel the contraction in the triceps muscle as you extend your arms.

Bent-over Triceps Kickback

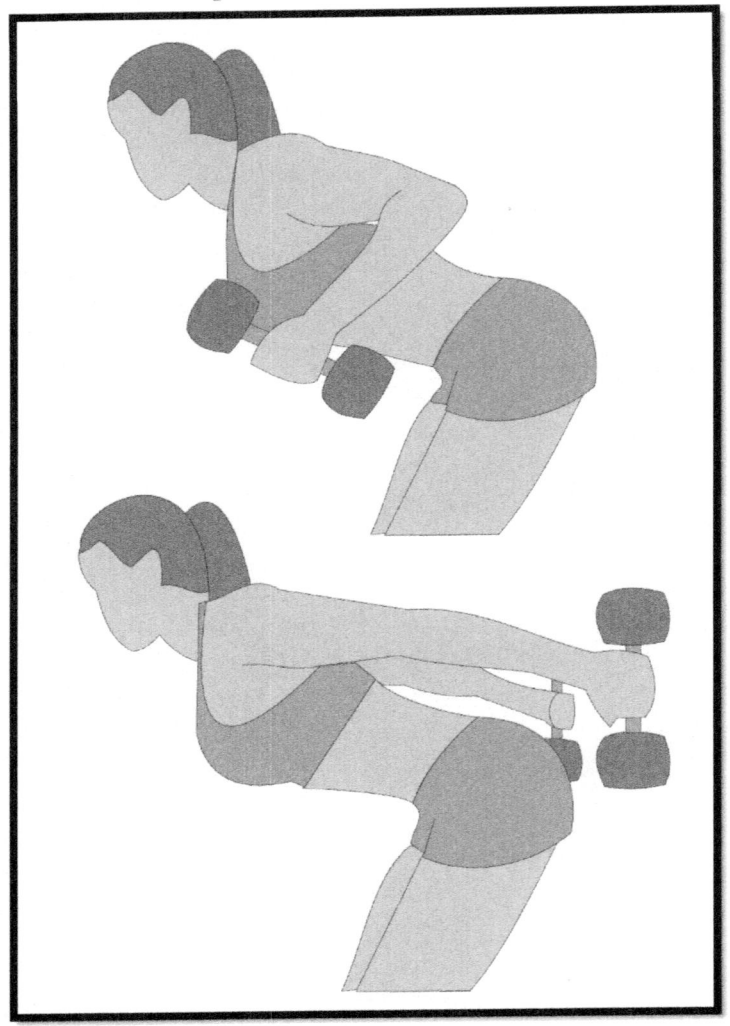

Strength Training with Dumbbells

Effect: This exercise mainly focuses on strengthening of the triceps muscles.

Difficulty Level: Intermediate

Start Position: Grab dumbbells in your hands facing the body and stand with feet hip width distance apart, knees slightly bent and torso bent at the waist almost parallel to the floor. Your upper arms should be close to your body, parallel to the floor and forearm pointing towards the floor holding dumbbells in the hands.

Steps:

1. Keeping your upper arms stationary straighten the lower arms taking dumbbells behind by contracting triceps.
2. Pause in the fully straighten position and slowly reverse the movement getting forearms to the start position.
3. Repeat required number of times.

Fine Tips:

1. The movement should be slow and controlled without momentum aiding in the movement.
2. Keep the upper arms steady all the time.

Shoulder Exercises

Seated Side Lateral Raise

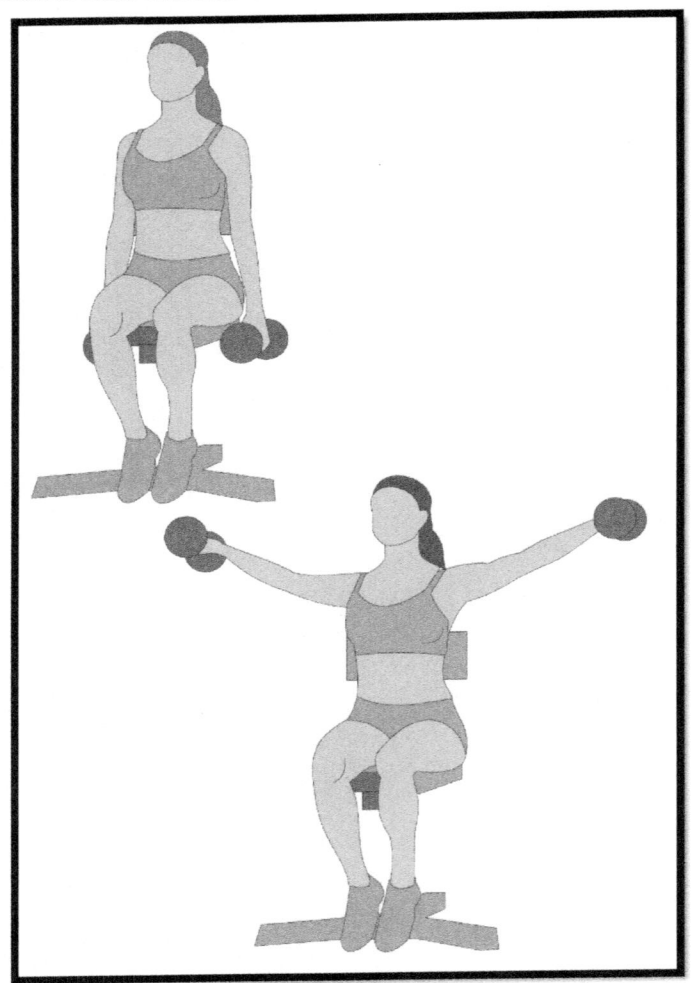

Strength Training with Dumbbells

Effect: This exercise strengthens muscles in the side of the shoulder, and upper back. Done with core engaged, it works on core stability.

Difficulty Level: Intermediate

Start Position: Grab the dumbbells with the palms facing inwards and arms by the side of the body and sit tall on the chair.

Steps:

1. Raise the dumbbells laterally from the start position up to the shoulder level, keeping the elbows slightly flexed.
2. Bring them back slowly to the start position.
3. Repeat required number of times.

Fine Tips:

1. Keep your neck tall, chin parallel to floor and core engaged throughout the movement.

Alternate Dumbbell Incline Bench Press

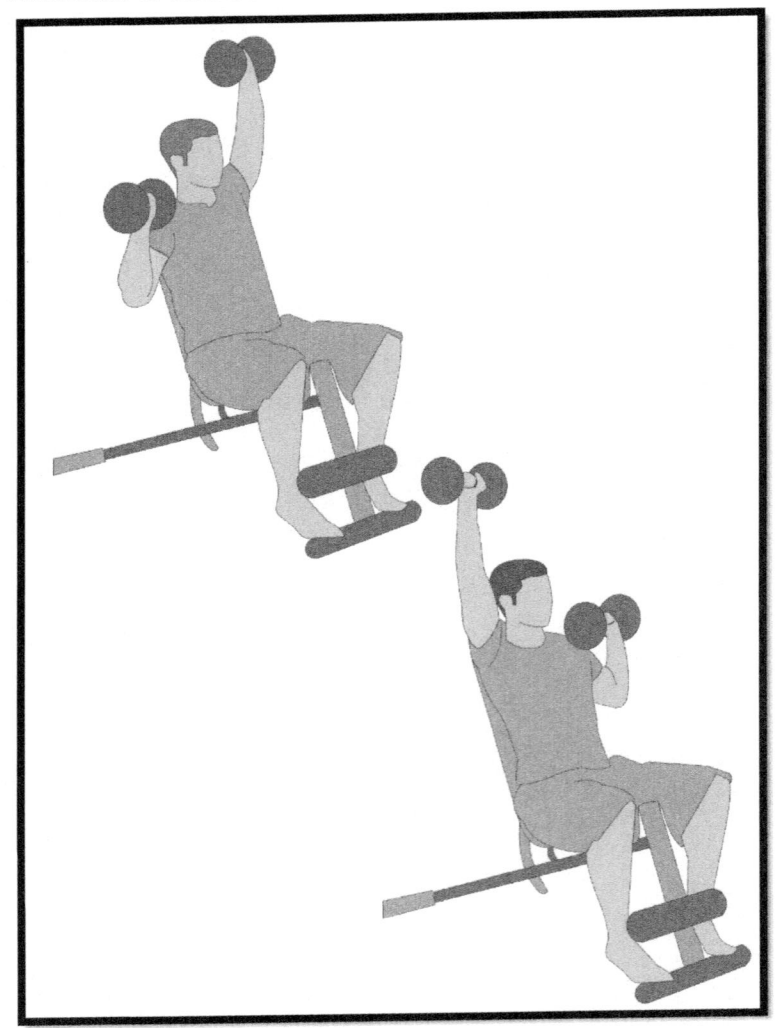

Strength Training with Dumbbells

Effect: This exercise helps to strengthen the shoulder, upper back and triceps muscles. The incline position of the bench increases the resistance on shoulder, upper back and chest.

Difficulty Level: Advanced

Start Position: Sit on the bench inclined at 45 degrees with the dumbbells held above your chest (sternum) and palms facing forward. Keep your feet firmly planted.

Steps:

1. Pull your shoulder blades together, slightly stick out your chest and lower the right dumbbell by the side of your chest.
2. Push the dumbbell to the start position as you lower the left dumbbell to the side of the chest.
3. Repeat alternatively on both the sides for required number of times.

Fine Tips:

1. Do not hyperextend your neck during the movement.
2. Keep your elbows close to your body throughout the movement.
3. Pause at the top of the press.

Dumbbell L-Arm Lateral Raise

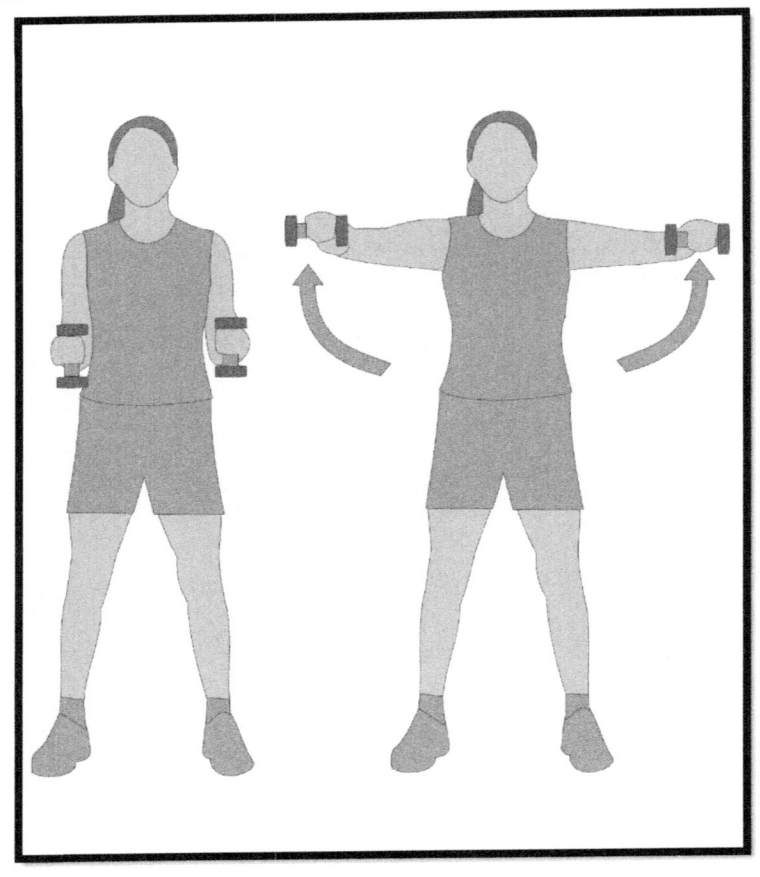

Strength Training with Dumbbells

Effect: This exercise focuses on strengthening of rotator cuff muscles and stability of scapular region. Performing this exercise in standing position actively engages your core.

Difficulty Level: Intermediate

Start Position: Grab dumbbells in your hands with palms facing each other and arms bent at 90 degrees at the elbows, resting by the side of your body.

Steps:

1. Raise your arms, rotating at the shoulder, till they come parallel to the floor.
2. Retract your scapula and pause in the top position.
3. Slowly return to the start position.
4. Repeat required number of times.

Fine Tips:

1. Do not raise your arms too high up.
2. Focus on the form.

Overhead Dumbbell Press

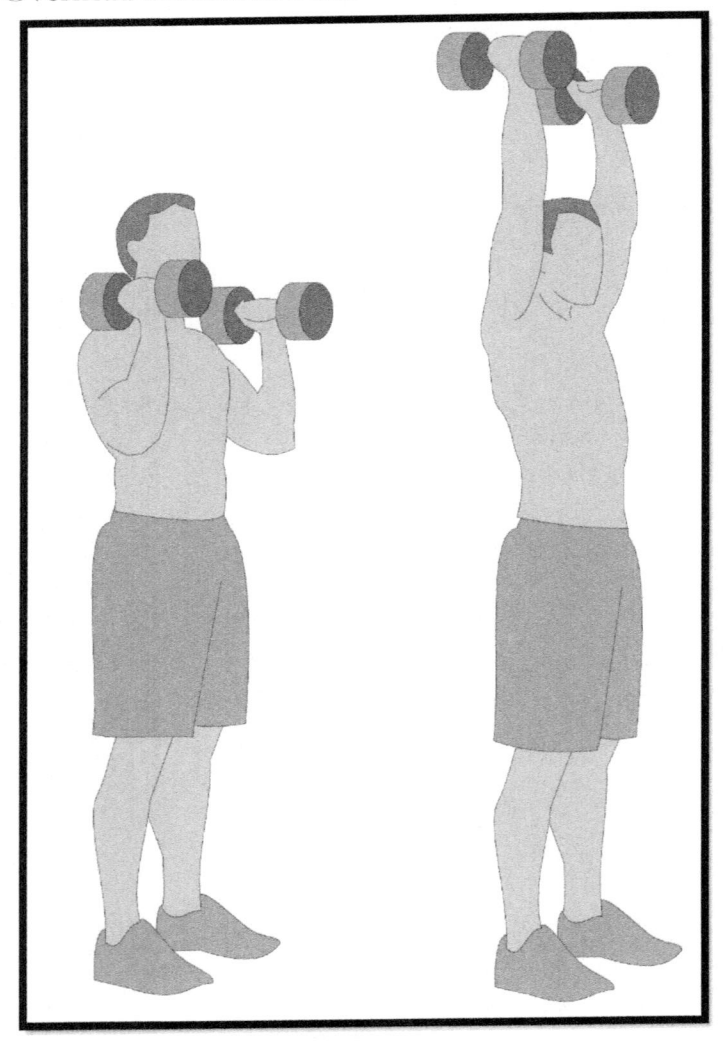

Strength Training with Dumbbells

Effect: This exercise works on the strengthening of arms and shoulder region. Exercise being done in the standing position keeps the core engaged throughout the exercise.

Difficulty Level: Beginner

Start Position: Grab the dumbbells outside your shoulders with your arms bent and palms facing each other. Stand tall with feet shoulder width apart.

Steps:

1. Raise your arms straight up till your arms are straight.
2. Pause and slowly lower the arms down to the start position.
3. Repeat for the required number of times.

Fine Tips:

1. Keep your shoulder blades back and down throughout the movement for shoulder stability.
2. Do not flare out the elbows during the movement.
3. Do not over arch your lower back as you push the dumbbells overhead.

Seated Overhead Dumbbell Press

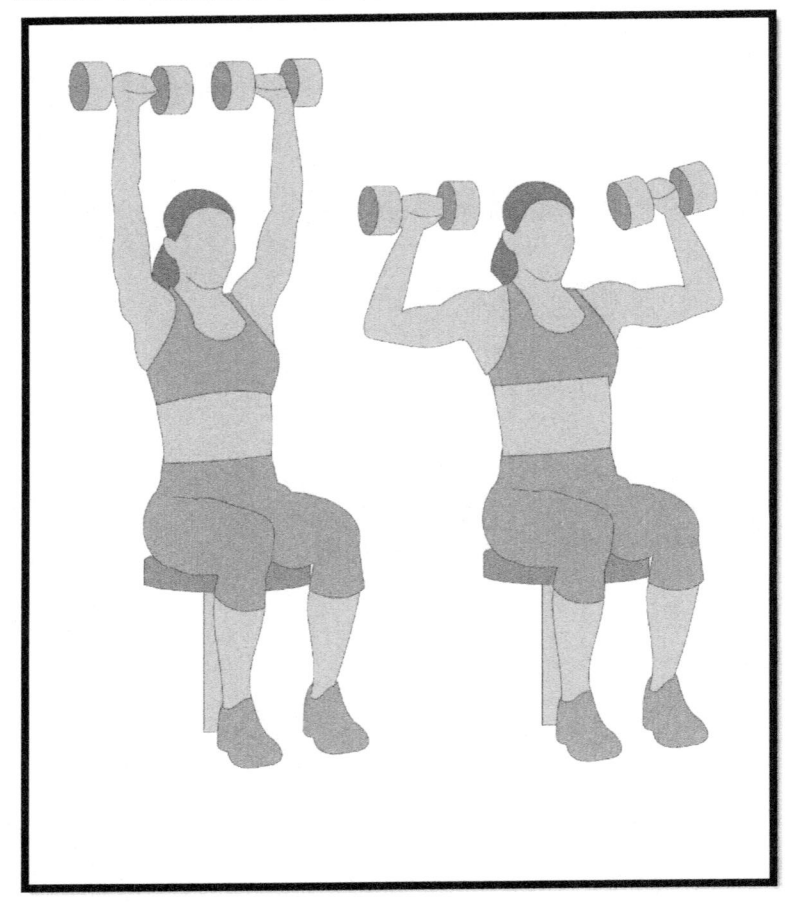

Strength Training with Dumbbells

Effect: This exercise strengthens the muscles in front of shoulder and on the back side of the arm.

Difficulty Level: Beginner

Start Position: Sit tall on a bench with your hips and knees at 90 degrees and feet grounded. Grab dumbbells in each hand at the shoulder level with elbows out and palms facing forward.

Steps:

1. Push the dumbbell overhead from the shoulder position till your arms are straight with palms facing forward.
2. Pause in the top most position and then lower down the dumbbells to the start position.
3. Repeat required number of times.

Fine Tips:

1. The movement should be slow and controlled.
2. In case of any discomfort in the shoulder region during movement, get the elbows closer to the body with palms facing each other.

Side Lying Lateral Raise

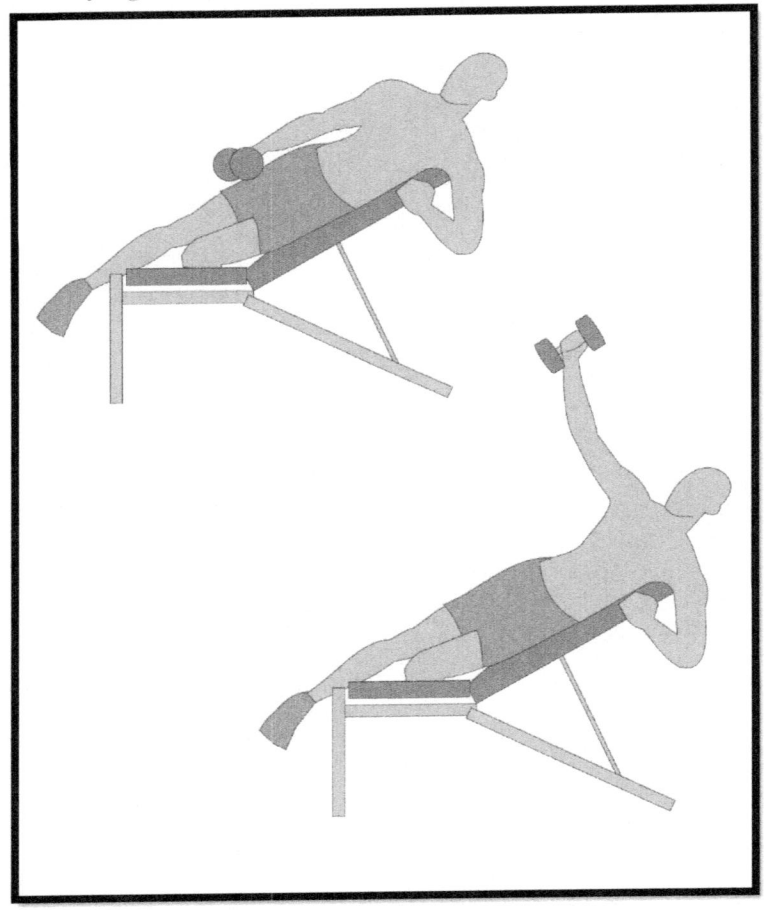

Strength Training with Dumbbells

Effect: This exercise helps to increase the strength and stability of the entire shoulder region focusing mainly on the muscles of lateral side of shoulder.

Difficulty Level: Intermediate.

Start Position: Grab a dumbbell in your hand and lie down on an inclined bench on the opposite side. The palm holding dumbbell should be facing the body with dumbbell resting on the side of upper leg.

Steps:

1. With the elbow slightly bent raise the dumbbell till the arm comes to 90 degrees with the upper body.
2. Slowly lower down the dumbbell to the start position.
3. Repeat for desired number of times.
4. Switch sides and repeat the sequence.

Fine Tips:

1. The movement should be slow and controlled. Avoid momentum aiding in the movement.

Dumbbell Pull Over the Head

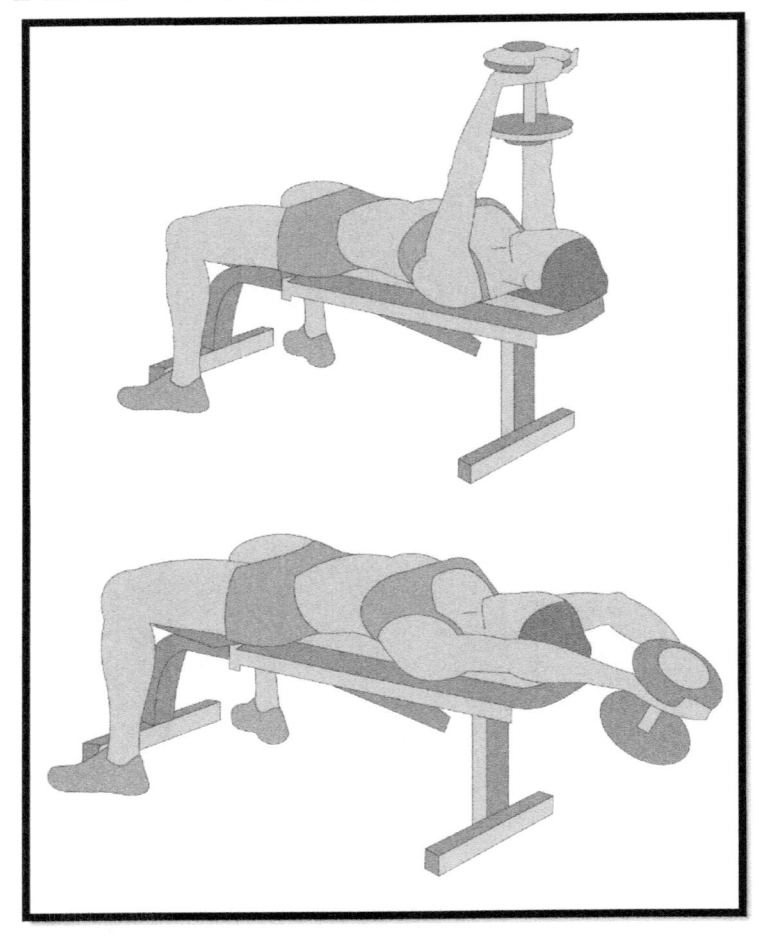

Strength Training with Dumbbells

Effect: This exercise strengthens the large muscles on both sides of the spine, back of the arm muscles and chest muscles.

Difficulty Level: Intermediate

Start Position: Lie down flat on your back on the bench with your feet firmly grounded. Make a grip with one hand over the other and grab a dumbbell from one edge with rest of the dumbbell hanging down. Hold the dumbbell with your arms straight above your chest.

Steps:

1. From the start position of the dumbbell, lower the dumbbell over your head till you feel a comfortable stretch in the chest region.
2. Pause and slowly reverse the movement.
3. Repeat the movement for required number of times.

Fine Tips:

1. Keep your core engaged by imprinting your lower back on the bench throughout the movement.
2. The movement should be slow and controlled.
3. Do not bend your elbow while lowering the dumbbell over your head.

Upright Row

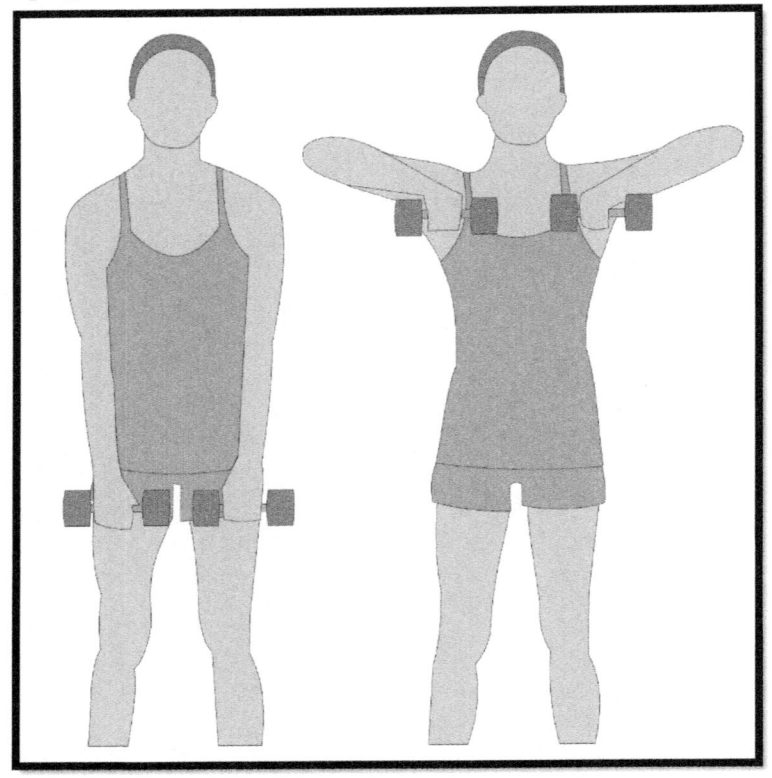

Strength Training with Dumbbells

Effect: This is a compound exercise that strengthens the back and shoulder muscles, specifically targeting trapezius and lateral deltoid.

Difficulty Level: Intermediate

Start Position: Stand tall and grab dumbbells in your hands in overhand grip at your thigh level with your palms facing your body.

Steps:

1. Raise the dumbbell straight up flaring out your elbows till the dumbbells reach your chest.
2. Hold dumbbells in the up position for a second.
3. Slowly reverse the movement and return to the start position.
4. Repeat required number of times.

Fine Tips:

1. The movement should be slow and controlled without the momentum aiding in the movement.
2. Keep the dumbbells close to your body all the time.
3. Do not shrug your shoulders as you raise the dumbbells.

Dumbbell Swing

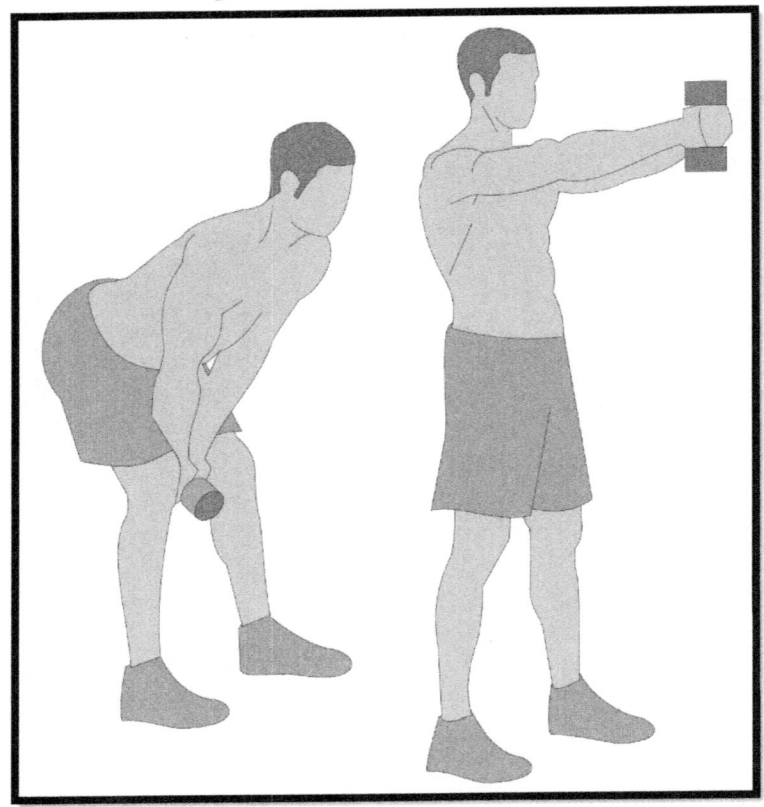

Strength Training with Dumbbells

Effect: This exercise helps to primarily strengthen the shoulder muscles. It also works to some extent on upper back, lower back and triceps muscles.

Difficulty Level: Intermediate

Start Position: Grab a dumbbell in both hands with fingers interlocked, between your legs and stand with feet little wider than shoulder width. The knees and hips should be slightly bent.

Steps:

1. Swing the dumbbell to the shoulder height straightening your legs and driving the hips forward as you straighten your back.
2. Slowly reverse the movement and return to the start position.
3. Repeat required number of times.

Fine Tips:

1. The exercise should be one fluid movement.
2. Bring down the dumbbell slowly.
3. Driving hip forwards is a must as you swing the dumbbell up.

Dumbbell Front Raise

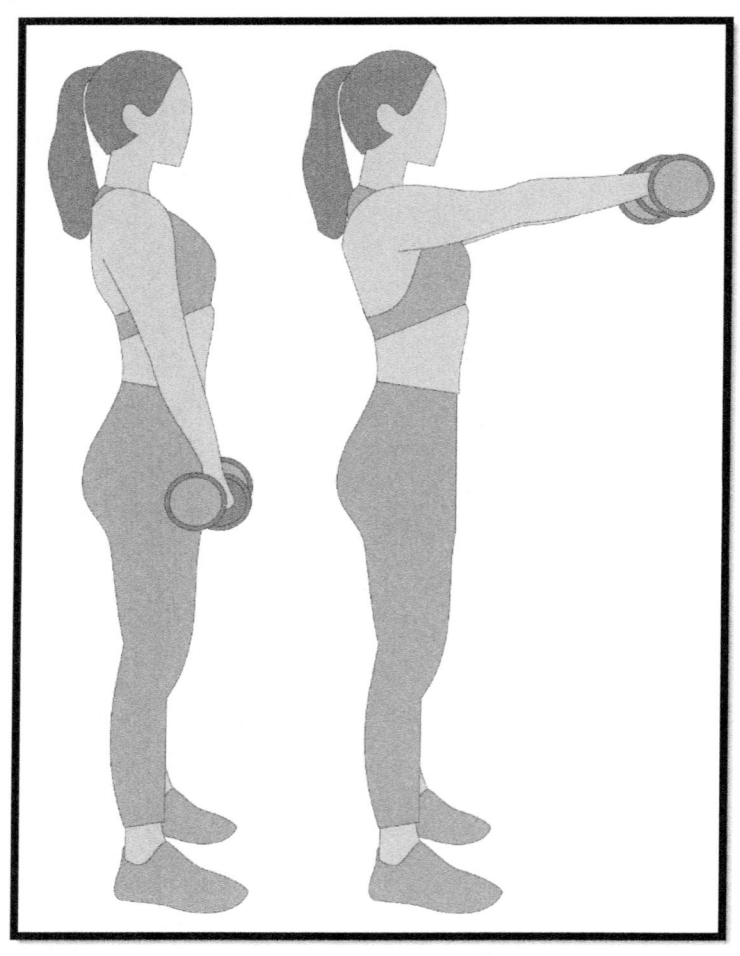

Strength Training with Dumbbells

Effect: This exercise mainly strengthens the shoulder muscles.

Difficulty Level: Beginner

Start Position: Grab the dumbbells with palms facing down, in front of your thighs and stand tall with feet shoulder width apart.

Steps:

1. Raise the dumbbells up, keeping the elbows slightly bent, so that the dumbbells reach at a level where arms are slightly higher than parallel to the floor.
2. Pause at the top and slowly reverse the movement.
3. Repeat required number of times.

Fine Tips:

1. Keep your torso straight throughout the movement.
2. The movement should be slow and controlled.

Dumbbell Shoulder Shrug

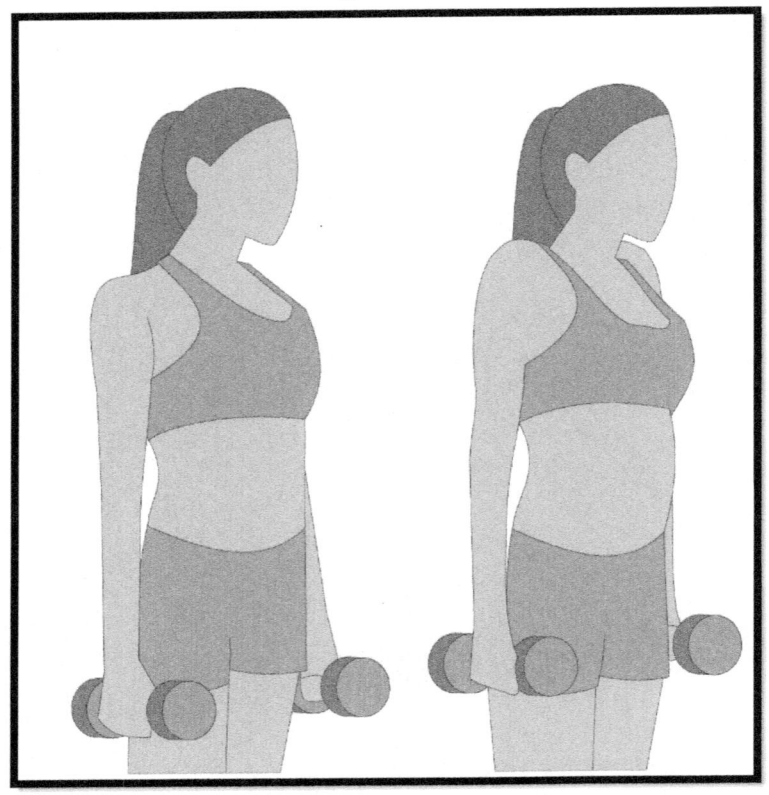

Strength Training with Dumbbells

Effect: This exercise strengthens the shoulder muscles.

Difficulty Level: Beginner

Start Position: Grab dumbbells by the side of your body with arms straight and palms facing the body. Stand with feet hip width distance apart and torso straight.

Steps:

1. Shrug your shoulders from the start position keeping your arms and torso straight.
2. Pause at the top position.
3. Slowly return to the start position.
4. Repeat required number of times.

Wrist Exercises

Seated Dumbbell Palm-up Wrist Curl

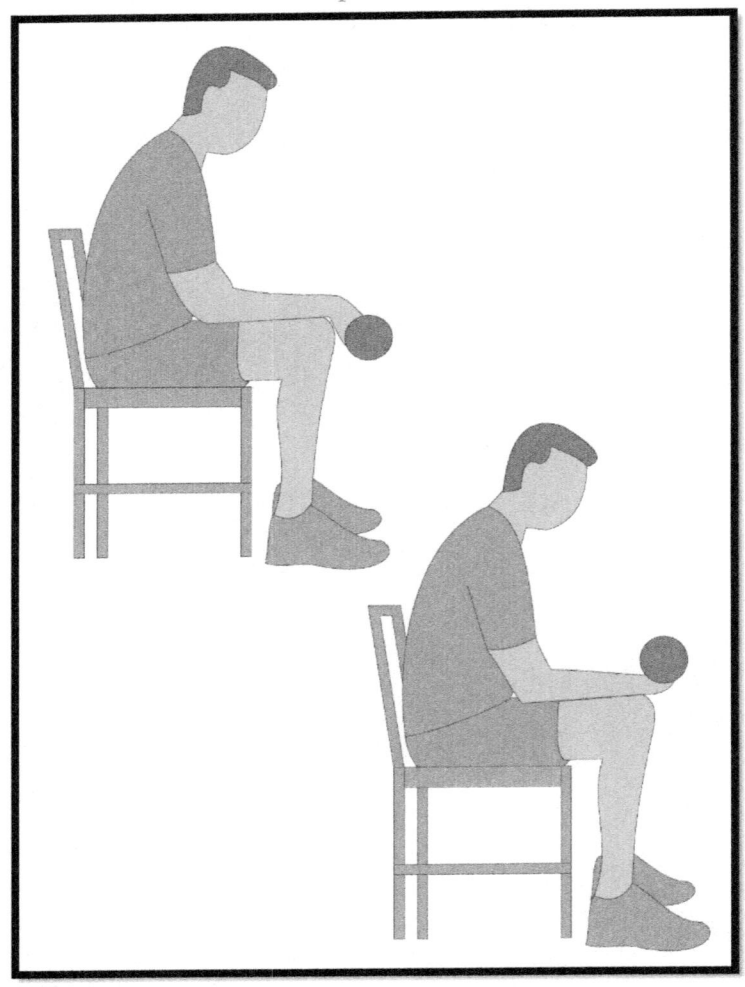

Strength Training with Dumbbells

Effect: This exercise focuses on strengthening of forearm muscles.

Difficulty Level: Beginner

Start Position: Sit on the chair with your feet hip distance apart and grounded. Grab two dumbbells in your hands, palm facing up, with your forearms resting on the thighs. The wrists should be hanging over the edge of your thigh.

Steps:

1. Start by curling your wrist up slowly using forearm muscles.
2. Slowly uncurl the wrist and reach the start position.
3. Repeat required number of times.

Fine Tips:

1. The movement should be slow and controlled.
2. Keep your arm and forearm stabilized throughout the movement.

Chest Exercises

Dumbbell Bench Press

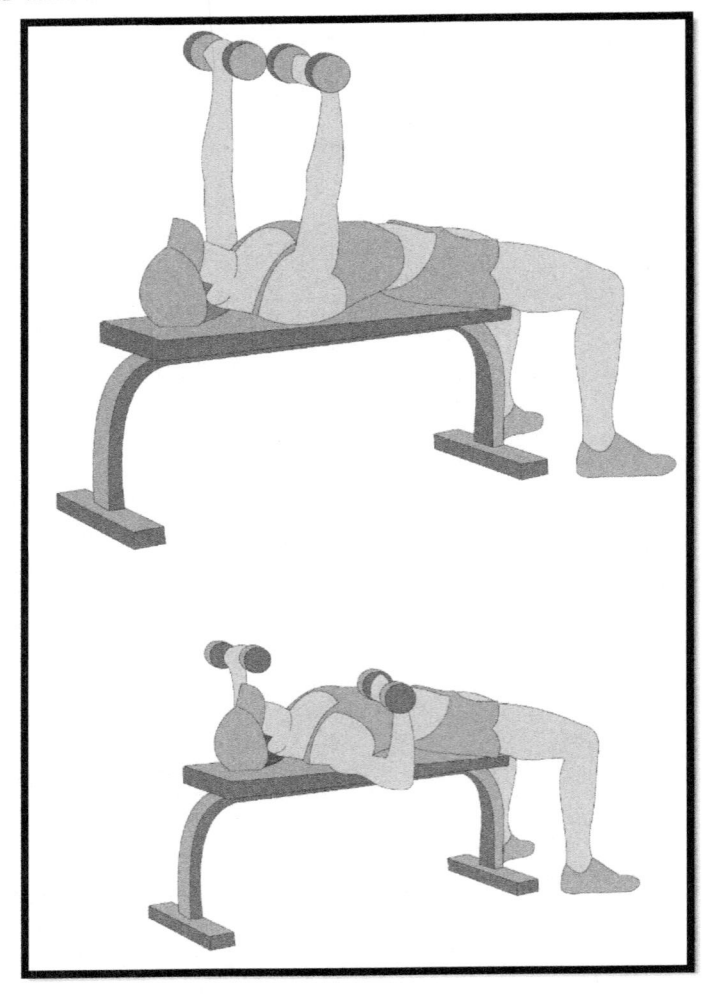

Strength Training with Dumbbells

Effect: This exercise helps in strengthening of shoulder, upper back, triceps and chest muscles with upper back in a supported position.

Difficulty Level: Intermediate

Start Position: Lie down straight on the bench with your feet placed firmly on the floor. Hold the dumbbells with arms extended, above your chest bone (sternum), palms pointing forward.

Steps:

1. Pull your shoulder blades together, slightly stick out your chest and lower the dumbbells towards the sides of the chest.
2. Pause near the chest and push the dumbbells back to the start position.
3. Repeat required number of times.

Fine Tips:

1. Do not hyperextend your neck during the movement.
2. Keep your elbows close to your body during the movement.
3. Pause at the top of the press.

Flat Dumbbell Crush Press

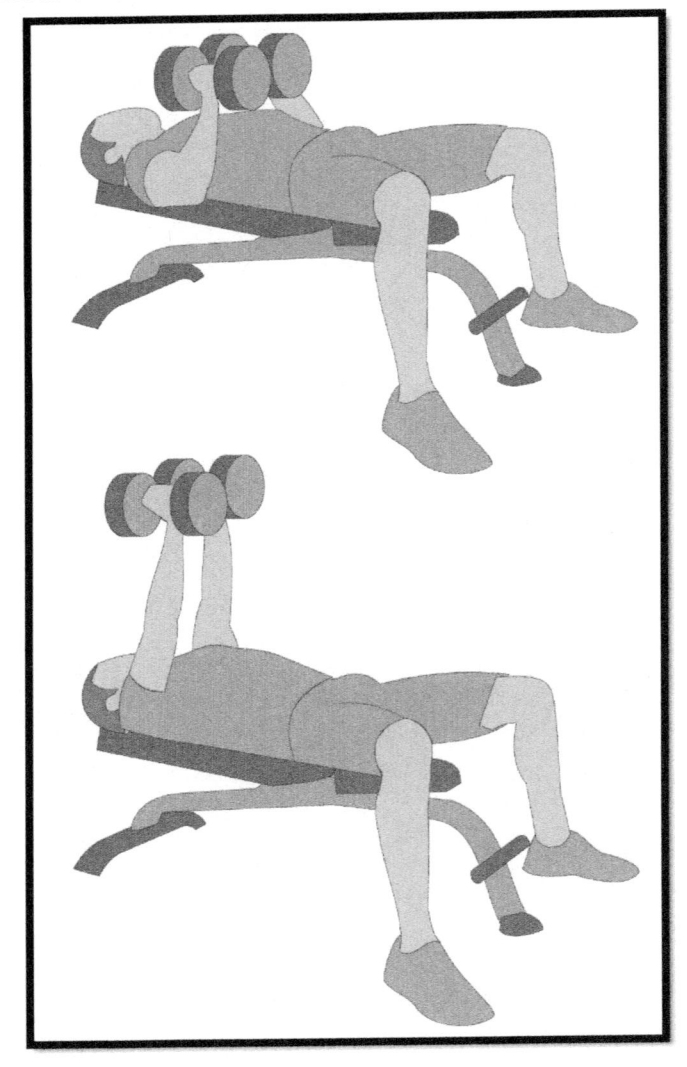

Strength Training with Dumbbells

Effect: This exercise helps to strengthen muscles in front of chest, front shoulder and back muscles of arm.

Difficulty Level: Intermediate

Start Position: Grab dumbbells in your hands with palms facing each other. Lie down flat on the bench with dumbbells over the chest, arms extended and feet placed firmly on the ground.

Steps:

1. Push the dumbbells against each other with arms in extended position.
2. Slowly lower the dumbbells to the middle of your chest by bending your arms, keeping them pressed against each other.
3. Reverse the movement returning to the Start Position.
4. Pause briefly at the top position and repeat again.
5. Do required number of repetitions.

Fine Tips:

1. Keep pressing the dumbbells against each other throughout the movement to increase muscle demand.

Incline Dumbbell Chest Fly

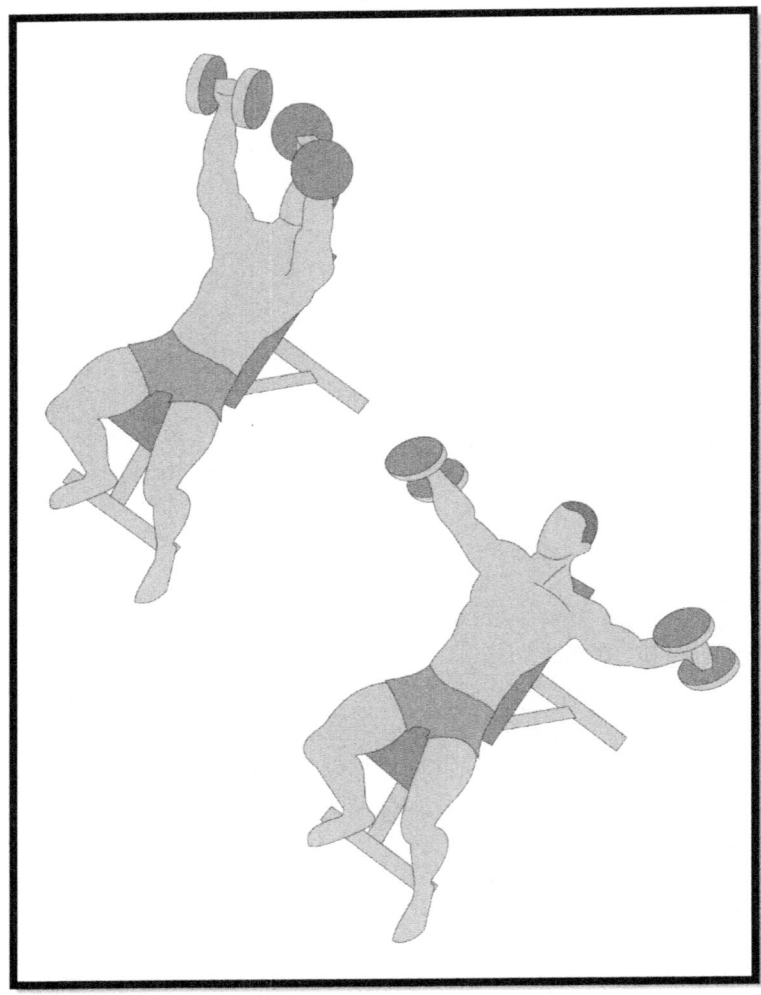

Strength Training with Dumbbells

Effect: This exercise strengthens the front muscles of your chest.

Difficulty Level: Intermediate.

Start Position: Lie down flat on a bench inclined at 45 degrees with feet firmly supported. Grab dumbbells with palms facing forward and arms extended over your chest.

Steps:

1. Keeping the arms soft at elbows and palms facing forward lower down the dumbbells to the side till you feel a slight stretch in the chest muscle.
2. Reverse the movement till your arms reach the start position.
3. Repeat required number of times.

Fine Tips:

1. The movement should be slow and controlled. Do not let momentum aid in the movement.

Dumbbell "T" Push-Ups

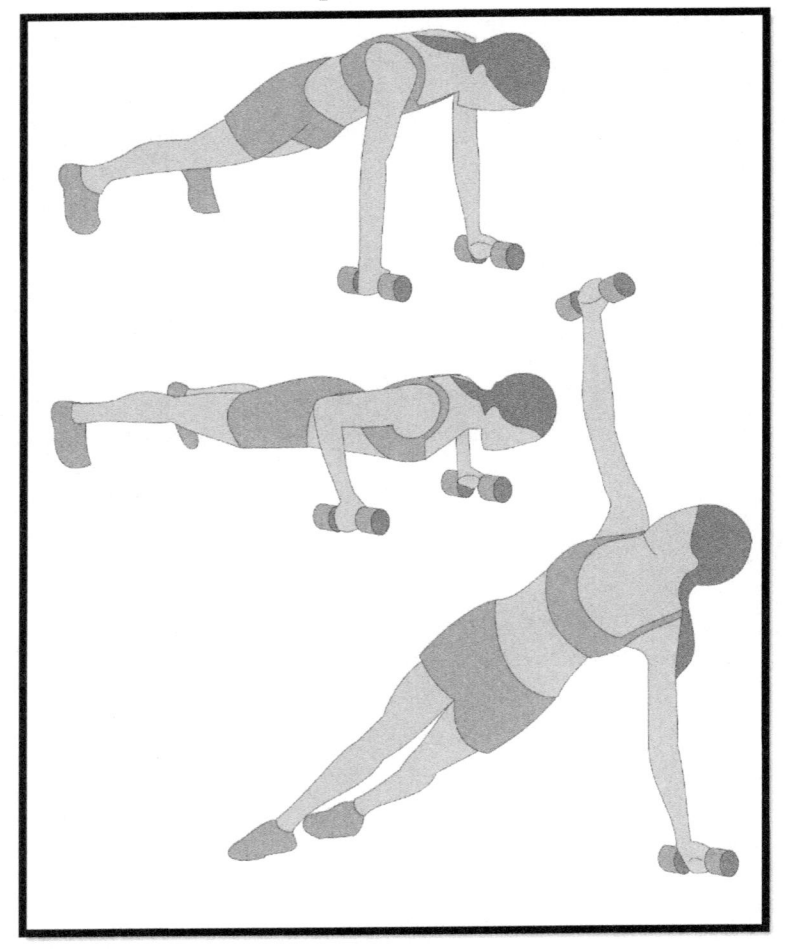

Strength Training with Dumbbells

Effect: This exercise mainly helps to strengthen the chest muscles and to some extent works out abs, glutes, shoulders, triceps, middle back and obliques too.

Difficulty Level: Intermediate

Start Position: Grab a pair of dumbbells and come in the push-up position with your hands slightly wider than the shoulder width and arms straight.

Steps:

1. Begin the exercise by lowering yourself down until your chest touches the floor.
2. Pause and then push yourself back up raising your right arm up as you rotate your body taking the right dumbbell up. Your right arm, shoulders and left arm comes in one straight line and body looks like "T" on its side with left side closer to the floor.
3. Reverse the movement back to the start position.
4. Repeat on the other side.
5. Repeat required number of times.

Fine Tips:

1. As you rotate the body, rotate your feet along with it. Keep your feet relaxed and do not force them to stay planted on the floor.
2. Raise arm straight up as you rotate.
3. Tighten your core throughout the movement.

Back Exercises

Dumbbell Rowing

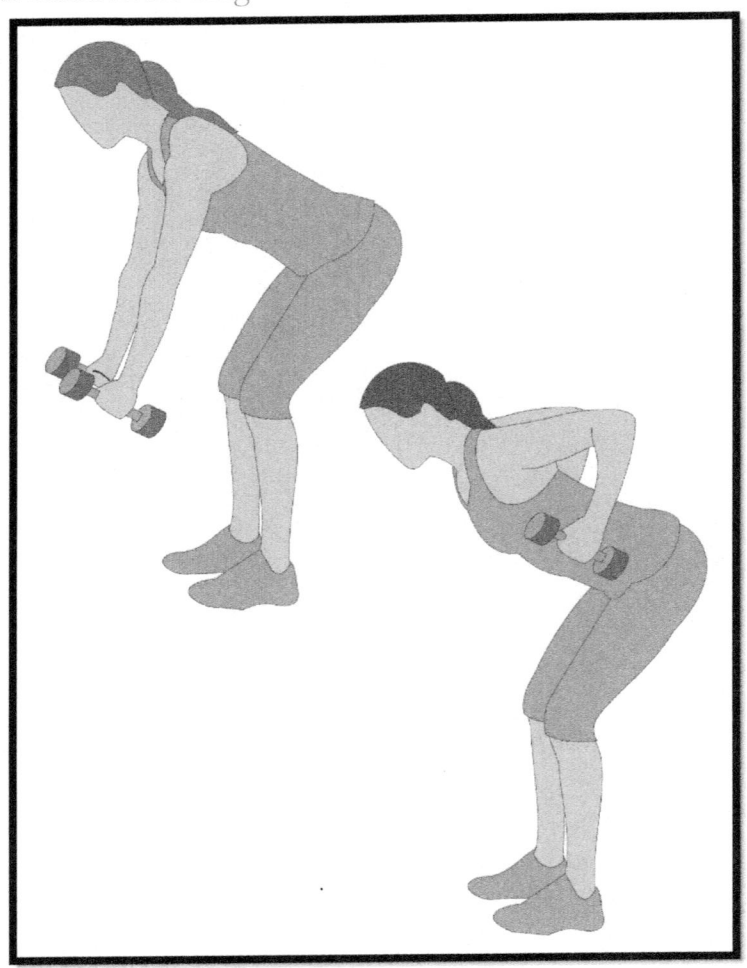

Strength Training with Dumbbells

Effect: This exercise works on strengthening of back, shoulder and biceps muscles along with increasing core stability.

Difficulty Level: Intermediate

Start Position: Grab dumbbells in both hands and stand with feet hip width apart, knees slightly bent, back tall and bent at the waist. Your hands should hang straight in front of your body.

Steps:

1. Retract the shoulders and bend the elbows raising dumbbells to the chest. Hold the dumbbells here for a second and then lower the dumbbells to the start position.
2. Repeat required number of times.

Fine Tips:

1. The movement should be controlled and slow.
2. Keep your core braced and back tall throughout the exercise.
3. Row the dumbbells to the side of your ribcage.

Renegade Row

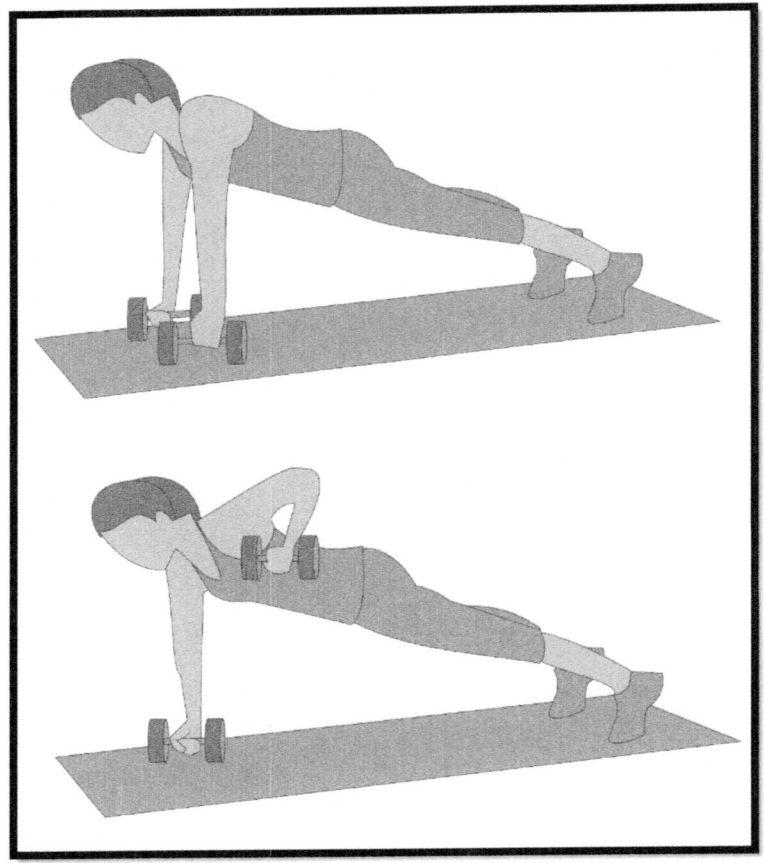

Strength Training with Dumbbells

Effect: This is a multiple joint exercise that increases strength in your back, biceps, triceps and shoulder muscles. Active engagement of core throughout the exercise works on core muscles also.

Difficulty Level: Intermediate

Start Position: Place the dumbbells at shoulder width distance apart and come in the push up start position with your hands grabbing the dumbbells.

Steps:

1. Row left dumbbell up towards the left side of your body while balancing on the right dumbbell and feet.
2. Pause on the top for a second and reverse the movement, getting dumbbell back to the start position.
3. Repeat on the other side. Do required number of repetitions.

Fine Tips:

1. Keep your body in straight line from shoulders to ankles throughout the movement.
2. Draw the scapula back together and do not slouch your back as you row the weight.

Supported Incline Chest Dumbbell Row

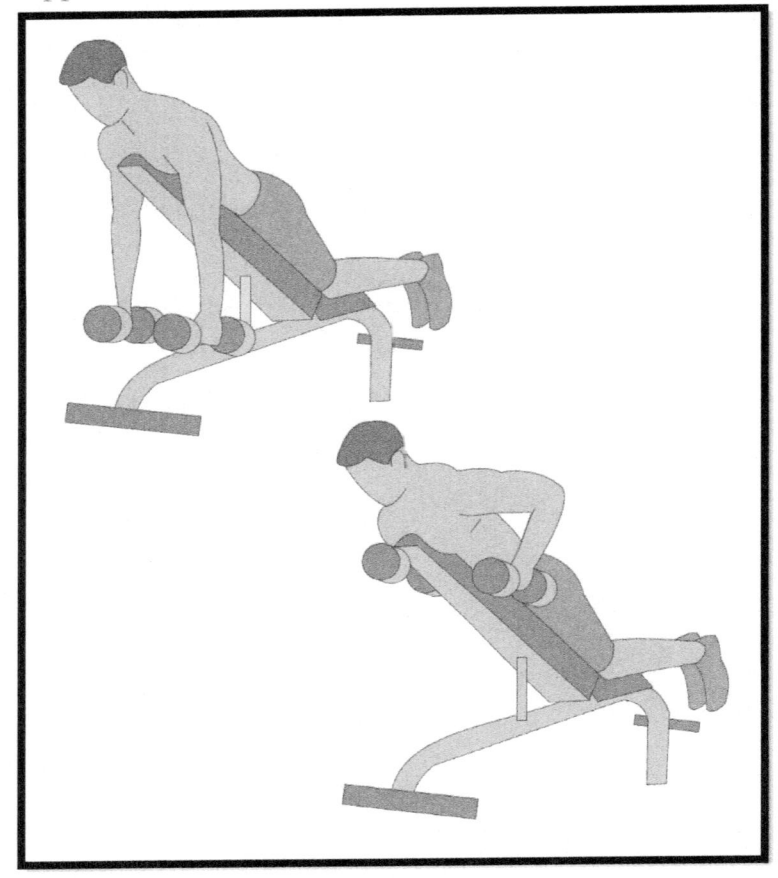

Strength Training with Dumbbells

Effect: This exercise mainly strengthens upper back, triceps and shoulder muscles.

Difficulty Level: Intermediate

Start Position: Lie down on a bench inclined at 45 degrees with your face down and head and upper chest hanging off the bench. Grab the dumbbells in your hands with palms facing each other and arms hanging straight down.

Steps:

1. Keeping your chest firm on the bench pad pull through your shoulder blades, bend your arms at elbows and pull them up till the dumbbells row to the bench level.
2. Reverse the movement and reach the start position.
3. Repeat required number of times.

Fine Tips:

1. Keep your chest firm on the bench. Do not use your back to aid in the movement.

Dr. Monika Chopra's Fitness Sutra

3-point Support Dumbbell Row

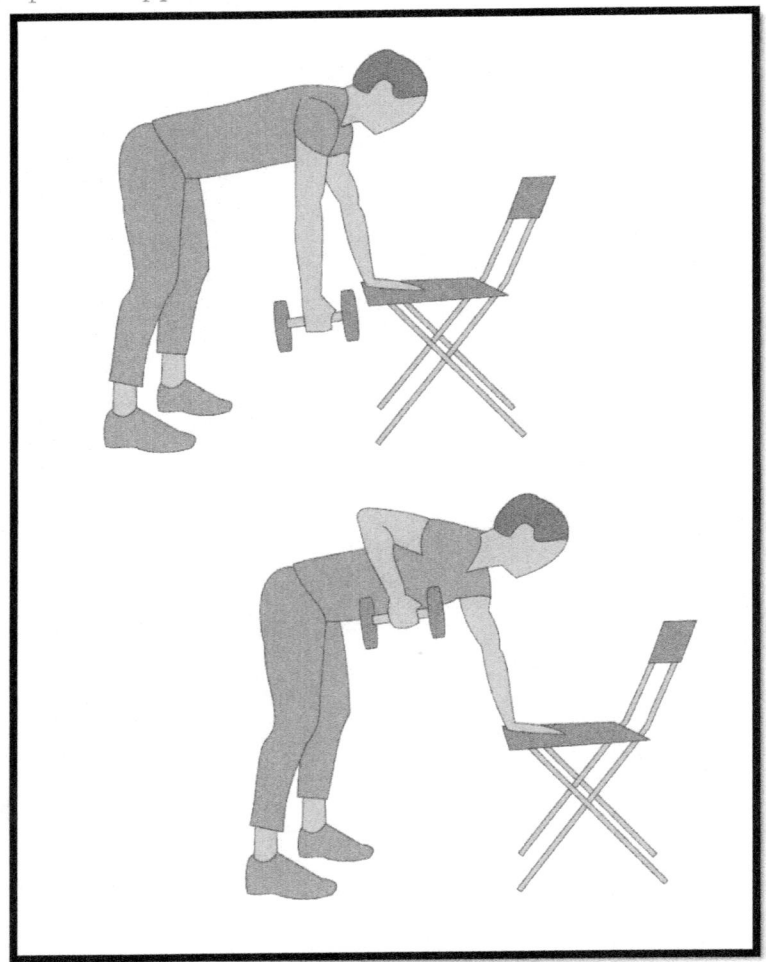

Strength Training with Dumbbells

Effect: This exercise strengthens the upper back muscles and muscles at the back side of the arms.

Difficulty Level: Intermediate

Start Position: Stand alongside facing a bench with feet hip width distance apart and bend at your waist planting your left hand at the bench keeping your upper back flat. Grab a dumbbell in your right hand with palm facing in and let the right arm hang straight down. Your feet and the left hand form the 3 support points.

Steps:

1. Pull your right shoulder blade to the middle and raise your right arm up bending at the elbow rowing the dumbbell till your chest level keeping your upper back flat and core engaged.
2. Pause at the chest level and slowly reverse the movement.
3. Repeat required number of times.
4. Switch the side and repeat on the other side.

Fine Tips:

1. Do not rotate the torso with movement. Keep your back flat and core engaged throughout the movement.

Bent-over Dumbbell Sideways Raise

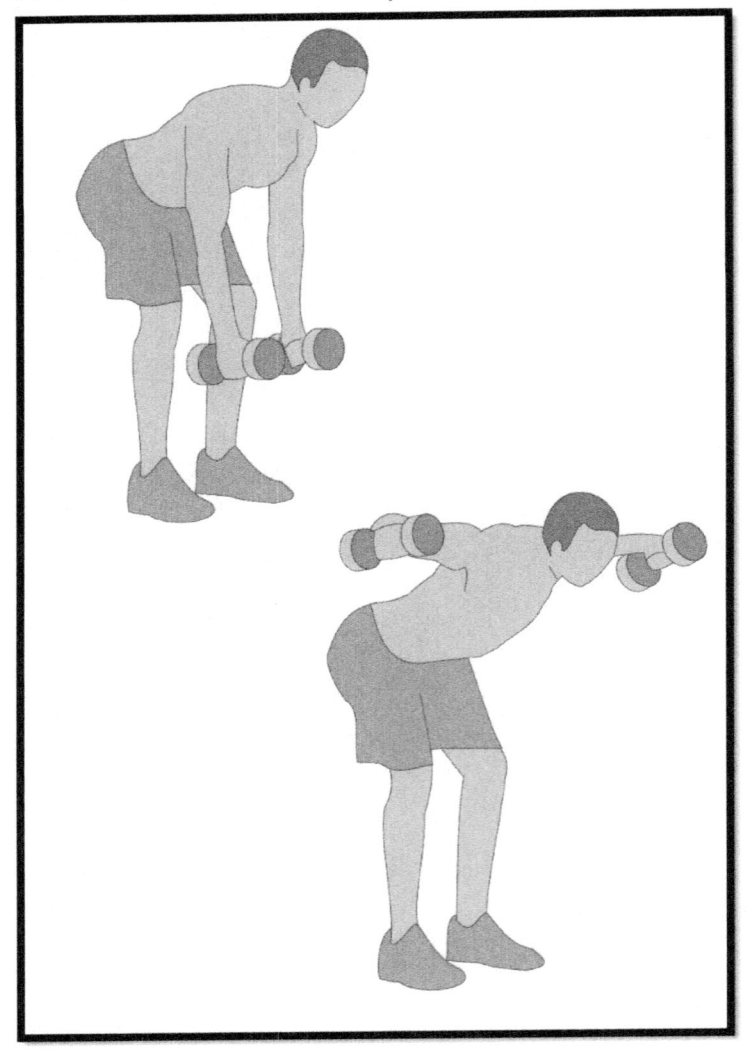

Strength Training with Dumbbells

Effect: This exercise helps to strengthen upper back muscles and muscles on the back side of the arm, especially posterior deltoid.

Difficulty Level: Intermediate

Start Position: Stand with feet hip width distance apart and bend at your waist keeping your neck and back parallel to the floor. Grab the dumbbells in your hands with palms facing each other and arms hanging straight down towards the floor.

Steps:

1. Using the upper back muscles and muscles at the back side of your arms, raise your arms sideways till they come parallel to the floor.
2. Pause and slowly lower down the arms to the start position.
3. Repeat required number of times.

Fine Tips:

1. Keep your neck aligned with your back and your back parallel to the floor throughout the movement.
2. The movement should be slow and controlled engaging your arms and back muscles.

Dr. Monika Chopra's Fitness Sutra

"You wake up in the morning, then go for a jog, pump up the dumbbell, and take a shower! Put on fresh and clean clothes and get out of your apartment fast! The day is yours for the taking! Carpe Diem!"

— Avijeet Das

CHAPTER 5

Lower Body Exercises

Quadriceps Exercises

Dumbbell Diagonal Lunge

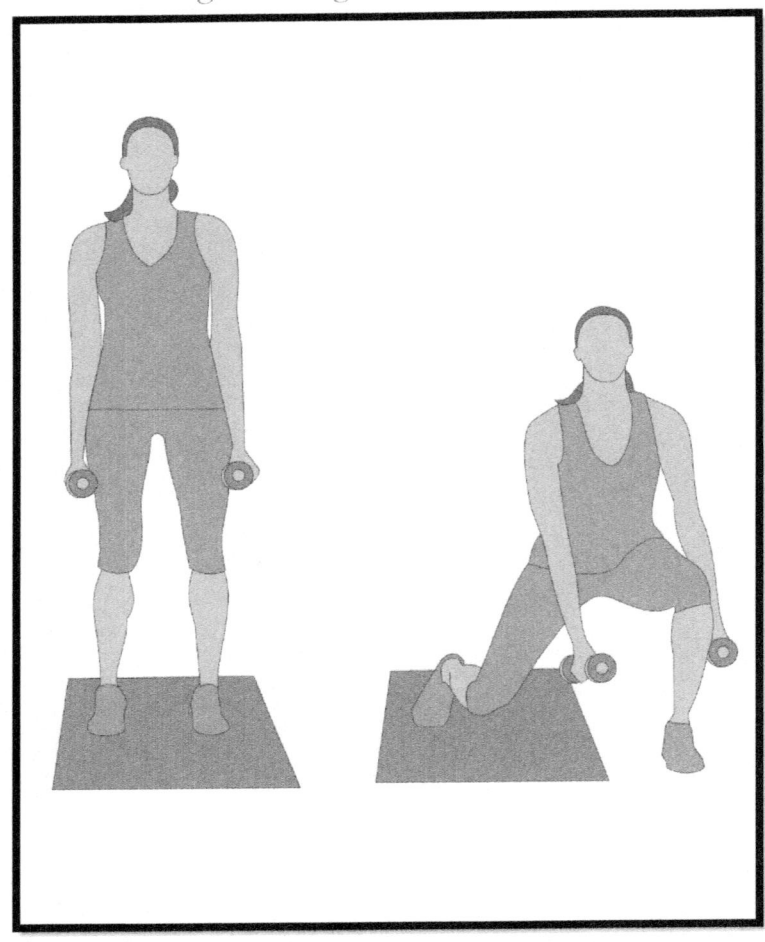

Strength Training with Dumbbells

Effect: Strengthening of quadriceps, gluteus and hamstring muscles. Improves lower body stability.

Difficulty Level: Intermediate

Start Position: Grab a pair of dumbbells with a neutral grip so that your palms are facing each other. Stand tall with your feet hip-width apart. Your arms should be hanging straight down by your sides.

Steps:

1. Take a large step forward diagonally at a 45-degree angle with the left foot, lowering your right knee toward the ground while keeping your left shin as vertical as possible.
2. Lower down till the left thigh becomes parallel to the floor
3. Pause here and push to the start position.
4. Do the required number of repetitions and repeat on the other side.

Fine Tips

1. The rear foot should not rotate instep as you lower down the body.
2. Lowering down into lunge should happen by lowering the hip, keeping front knee over the ankle.

Walking Dumbbell Lunge

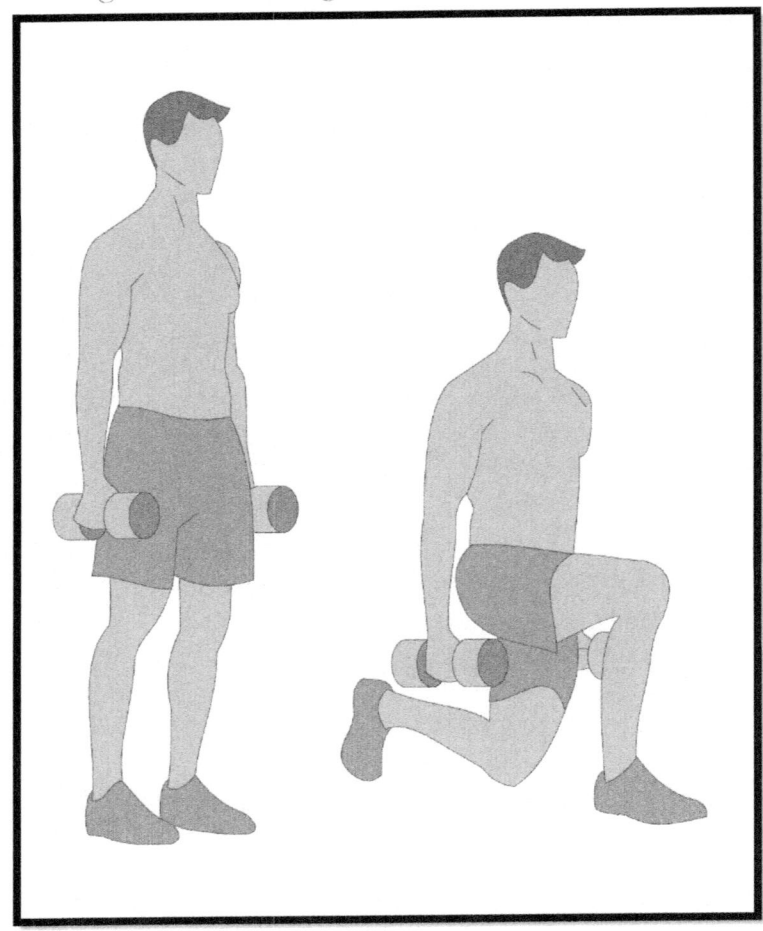

Strength Training with Dumbbells

Effect: Muscle strengthening of lower part of the body focusing on hams and gluteus muscles.

Difficulty Level: Intermediate

Start Position: Hold the dumbbells in a neutral position with arms straight by the side of your body and palms facing each other.

Steps:

1. Drop into a lunge with both knees at 90 degrees keeping your hips and shoulders squared (facing forwards) and back tall.
2. Step forward with your back leg bringing both feet together. Repeat movement with the opposite side.
3. Take required number of steps.

Fine Tips:

1. Centre your body weight on heel of the front foot.
2. Keep your back tall and shoulder squared all the time.
3. Take big enough steps so that your knees are always at 90 degrees.

Dr. Monika Chopra's Fitness Sutra

Dumbbell Lunge and Rotation

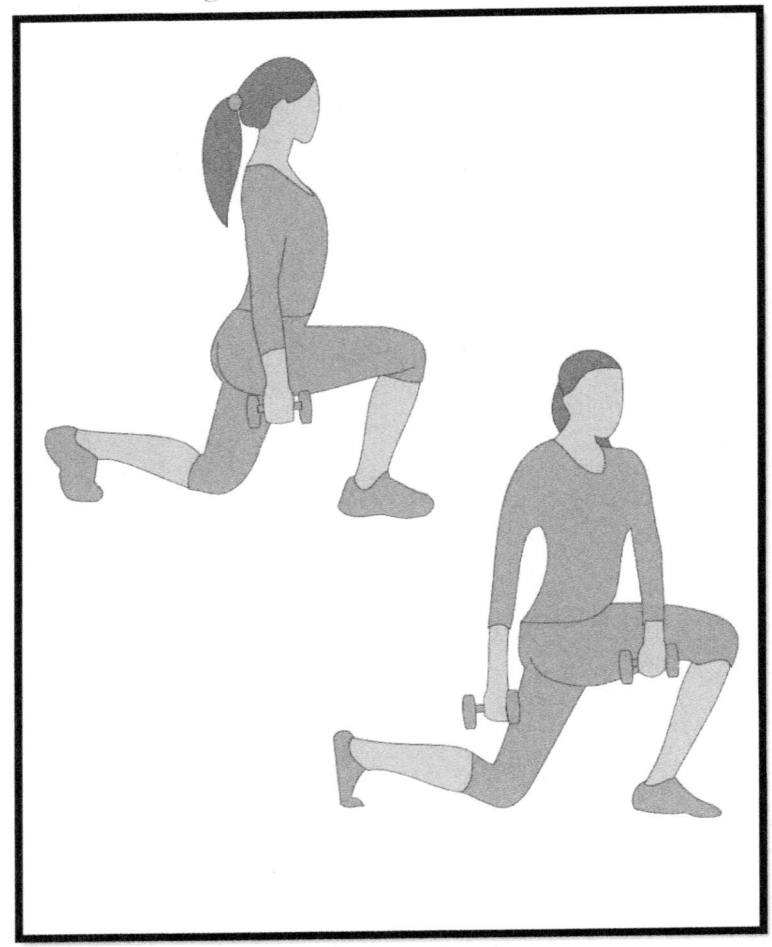

Strength Training with Dumbbells

Effect: This strengthening exercise targets hamstring, gluteus and quadriceps muscles. The rotational component works on improving core strength and stability.

Difficulty Level: Advanced

Start Position: Grab the dumbbells by the side of your body with palms facing each other. Step into the lunge position with rear knee on the floor and front knee at 90 degrees.

Steps:

1. From the start position rotate your torso so that the opposite arms rest on the outer side of the front bent leg.
2. Return to the start position.
3. Repeat required number of times.
4. Repeat on the other side.

Fine Tips:

1. Descend into lunge by dropping the hips down rather jutting the knee forward.
2. The rotation should start from abdomen to chest and then shoulder.
3. Keep the core braced and torso tall throughout the movement.
4. The knee should not cave inward with rotation.

Dumbbell Step

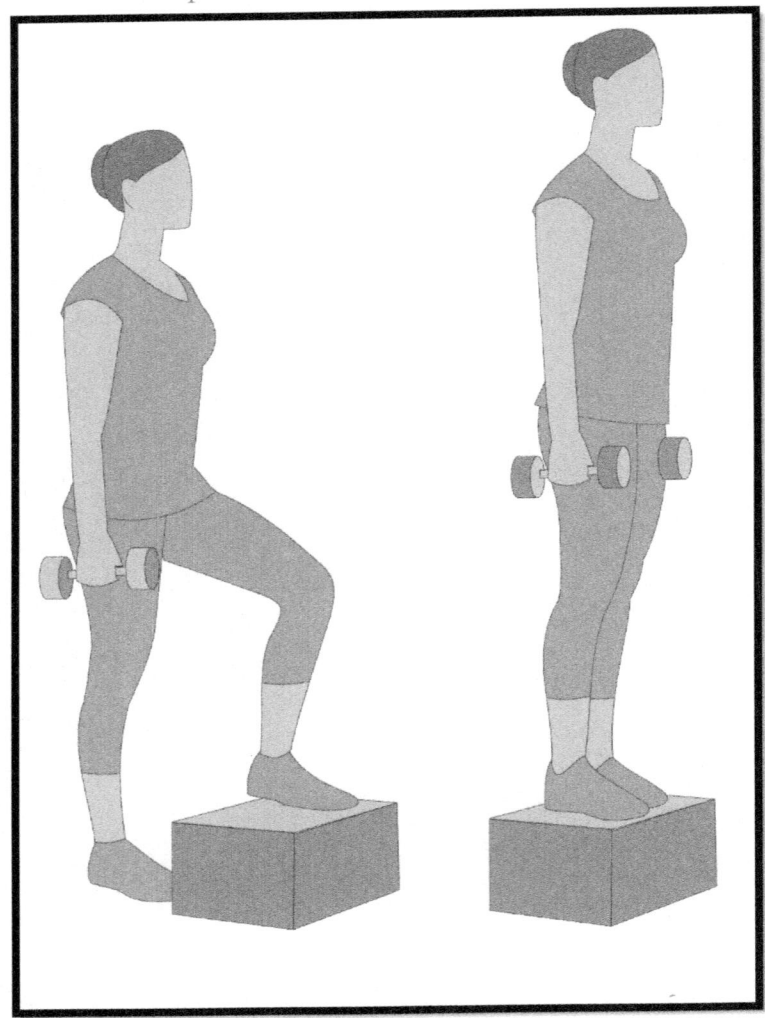

Strength Training with Dumbbells

Effect: Strengthening of gluteus, hamstring and quadriceps muscles. Increases core stability.

Difficulty Level: Beginner

Start Position: Grab dumbbells in your hands and stand tall with your feet hip width distance apart, shoulders and hips squared.

Steps:

1. Step on the platform from the start position taking your weight on the stepping foot by pressing through it and raise onto the platform.
2. Push your hips back and land on the floor on the support foot.
3. Repeat required number of times.
4. Repeat on the other side.

Fine Tips:

1. Stand tall as you raise onto the platform and back.
2. Never let your knee fall in as you step onto the platform and back to the floor.
3. Do not use the supporting leg to push you on the platform. Use the stepping foot to raise you instead.
4. Keep the stepping foot nicely planted on the platform as you step.

Side Lunge Jump off

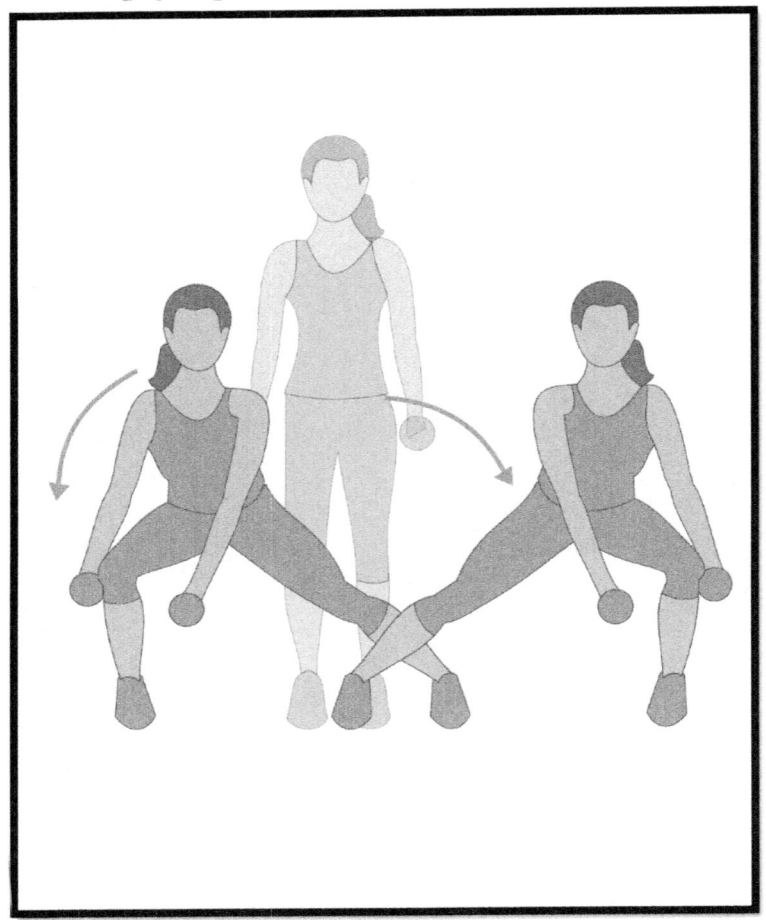

Strength Training with Dumbbells

Effect: This is a dynamic exercise that works on the strengthening of gluteus, hamstring and quadriceps muscles.

Difficulty Level: Intermediate

Start Position: Grab dumbbells in both the hands and stand in a side lunge position with right thigh parallel to the floor and right knee at 90 degrees. Dumbbells hang by the sides of the right knee.

Steps:

1. Jump and switch the leg coming in side lunge to the left side, hanging dumbbells by the side of the left leg.
2. Repeat the above sequence for required number of times.

Fine Tips:

1. Jump as high and far to the side as possible.
2. Avoid curving your back throughout the exercise.
3. Keep your weight centred on the back heel to help in lateral jump.

Dr. Monika Chopra's Fitness Sutra

Goblet Squat with Pulses

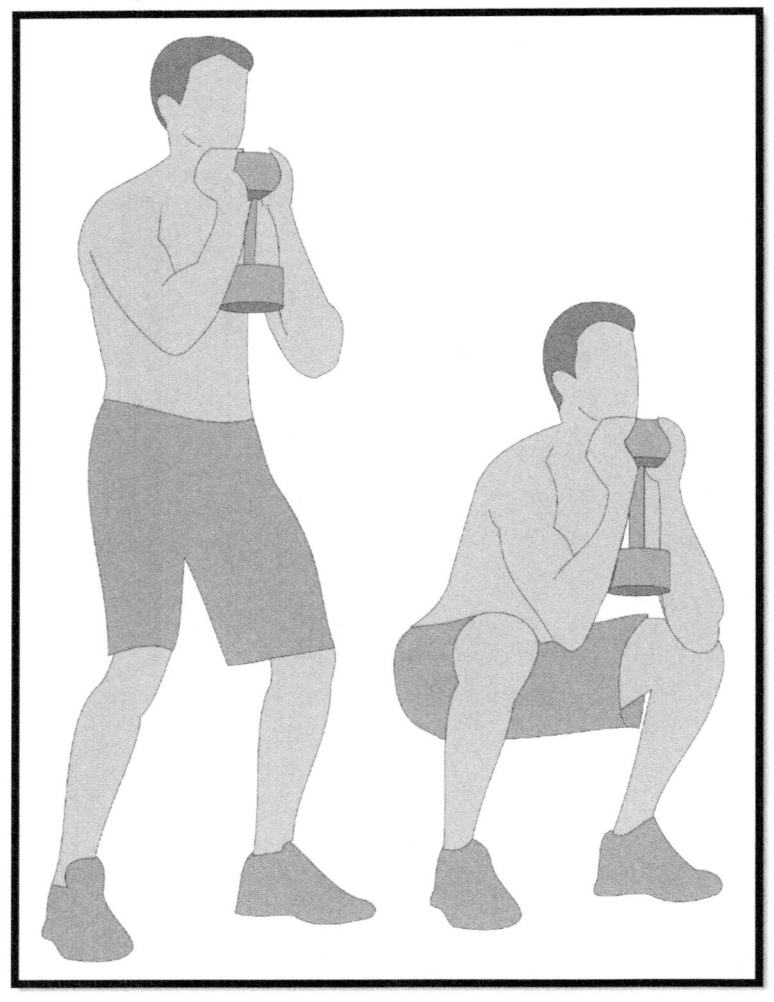

Strength Training with Dumbbells

Effect: This exercise primarily strengthens the quadriceps and also to lesser extent hamstrings, groin muscles, hip flexors, outer thighs and gluteus muscles.

Difficulty Level: Beginner

Start Position: Hold a dumbbell with both hands under your chin. Stand with your feet about shoulder width apart and your toes angled outwards.

Steps:

1. Bend at your knees and squat till your knees are slightly lower than 90 degrees.
2. Pulsate up and down about an inch a couple of times and then stand back to start position.
3. This completes one repetition.
4. Repeat required number of times.

Fine Tips:

1. Don't squat too much below 90 degrees.
2. Stay balanced and don't hunch over.
3. Focus on the stretch as you pulsate.

Dr. Monika Chopra's Fitness Sutra

Curtsy Lunge

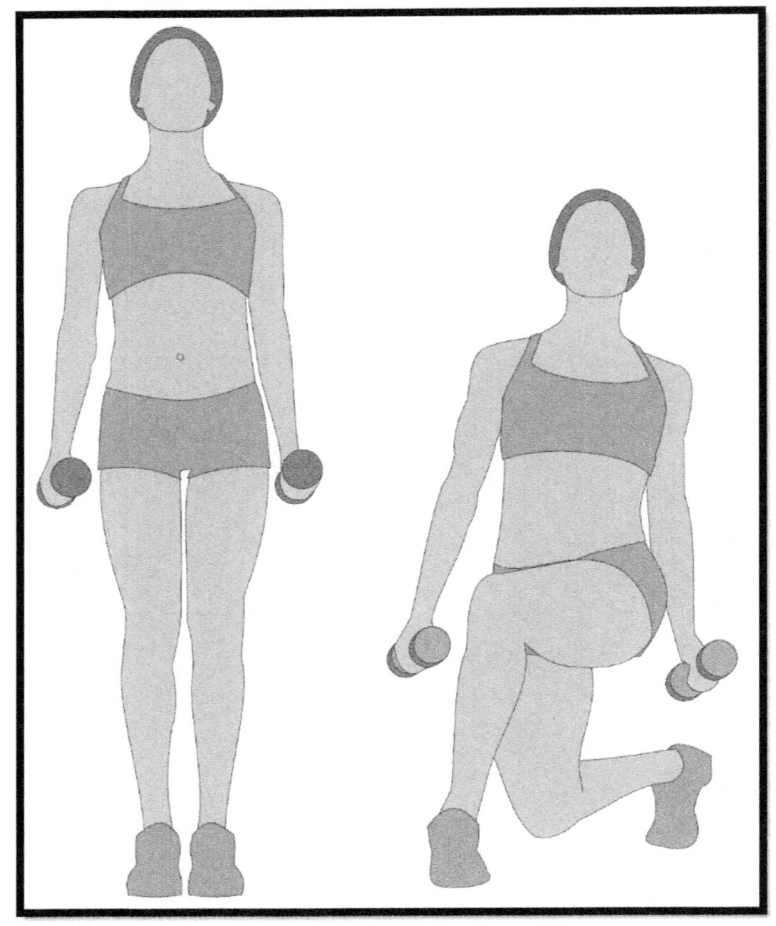

Strength Training with Dumbbells

Effect: This exercise mainly strengthens quadriceps muscles and also to some extent hip adductors, hip flexors, hamstrings, gluteus, groin muscles and calves.

Difficulty Level: Beginner

Start Position: Grab dumbbells in your hands with arms hanging straight down by the side of your body. Stand tall with shoulders and hips squared (pointing forwards) and chin parallel to the floor.

Steps:

1. Initiate the movement by shifting your weight to the left leg. Lift your right foot, keeping your torso facing forward, and place it diagonally behind the left foot with a long step.
2. Descend into the lunge by bending your knees, lowering your body straight down, till your knees are bent at 90 degrees and left thigh is parallel to the floor.
3. Drive through your heel, extend your hips and knees, and take your right foot to the start position.
4. Switch the leg and repeat on the other side.
5. Repeat required number of times.

Fine Tips:

1. Keep your hips and shoulders squared (facing forward) and back tall throughout the movement.

Bulgarian Split Lunge

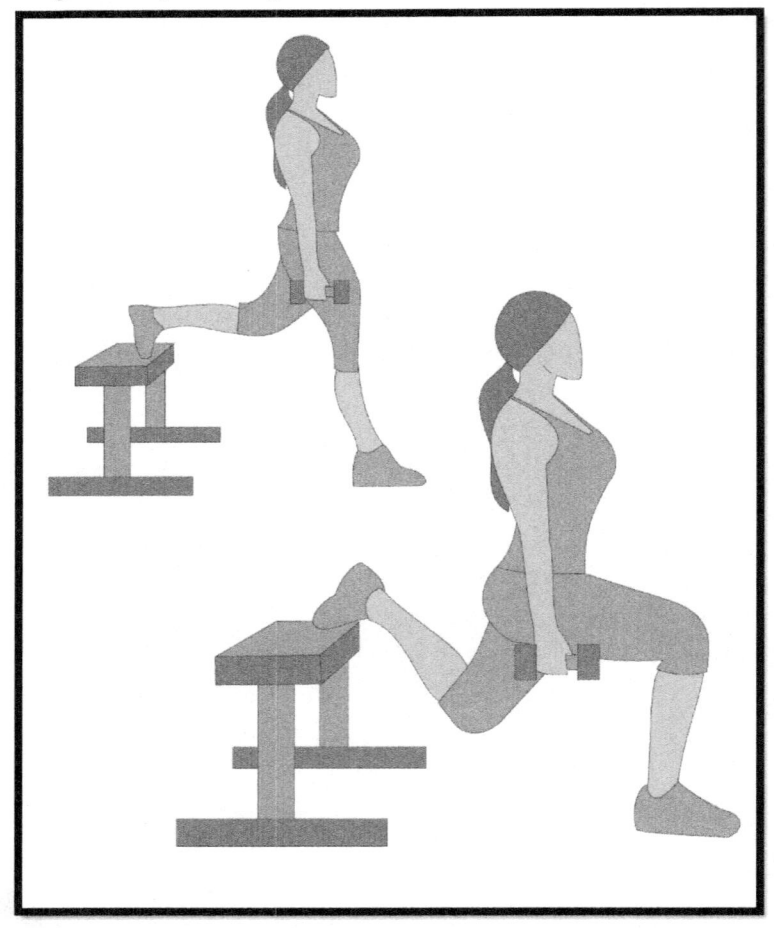

Strength Training with Dumbbells

Effect: This is a single leg strengthening exercise targeting quads, glutes and hamstring muscles. Performing exercise with dumbbells ensures muscle balance on both sides.

Difficulty Level: Intermediate

Start Position: Grab the dumbbells with your palms facing the body and arms hanging straight by the side of your body. With your feet hip width apart, place the instep of your left foot behind on a bench keeping a distance of 3 feet between both the feet.

Steps:

1. Lower your hips towards the floor so that the left knee comes closer to the floor and the right knee bends at 90 degrees.
2. Drive through the front heel and push back to the Start Position.
3. Repeat required number of times.
4. Switch the legs and repeat on the other side.

Fine Tips:

1. Do not let your front knee cave in as you lower down the hips.
2. Keep your hips and shoulders squared (facing forward) throughout the movement.
3. Make sure you descend into the squat position by lowering down the hips rather than jutting the knee forward.

Hamstring Exercises

Romanian Deadlift

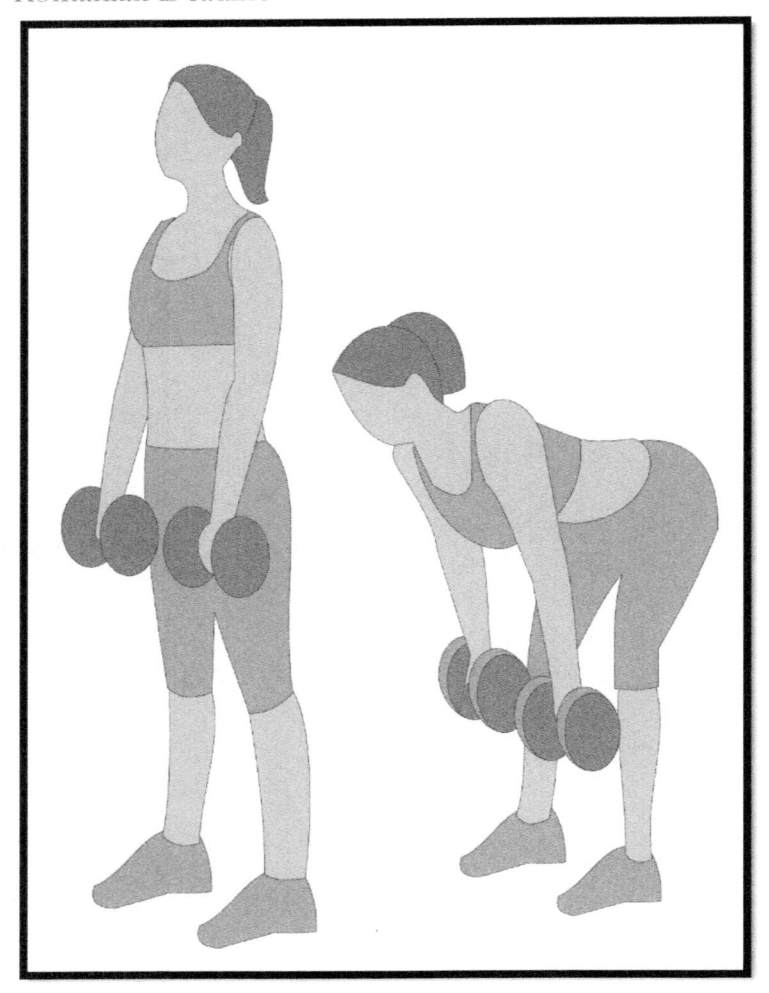

Strength Training with Dumbbells

Effect: This exercise helps to strengthen mainly hamstrings and to lesser degree glutes, hip flexors and lower back muscles.

Difficulty Level: Intermediate

Start Position: Stand tall with feet hip width distance apart and place dumbbells in front of feet.

Steps:

1. Bend over and pick up the dumbbells keeping your core tight and back straight.
2. Keep your knees slightly bent and use your hamstrings to pull your hips forward to standing and dumbbells to waist height.
3. Reverse the movement and lower the dumbbells straight down by hinging your hips till you feel slight stretch in hamstrings.
4. Repeat required number of times.

Fine Tips:

1. You don't have to lower the weight down to the floor all the time.
2. Use your hamstrings or hip muscles to lift and lower the weight and not arm muscles.
3. Keep your core tight and do not round the back during movement.

Single Leg Dumbbell Deadlift

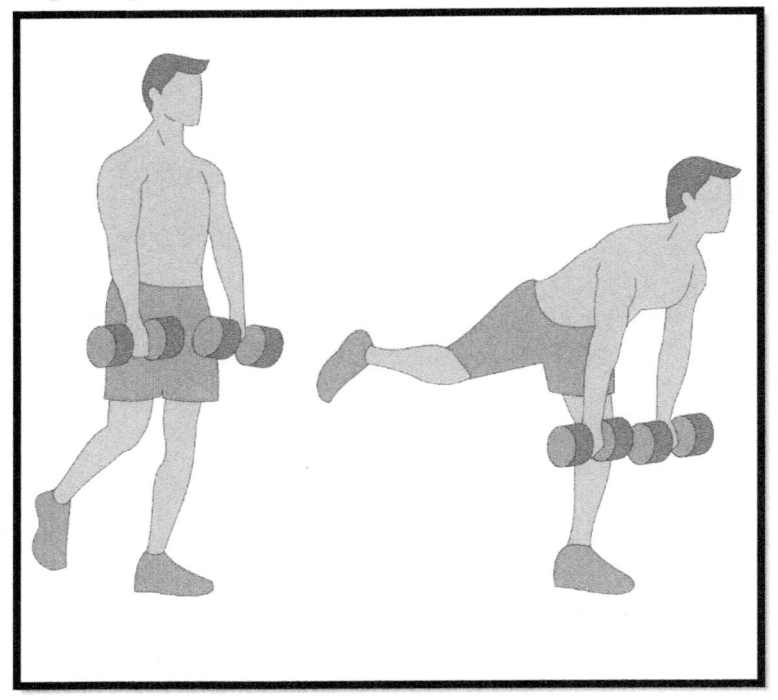

Strength Training with Dumbbells

Effect: This exercise mainly strengthens the hamstrings and to some degree quadriceps, lower back and calf muscles.

Difficulty Level: Intermediate

Start Position: Grab dumbbells in your hands by the side of your body and stand tall.

Steps:

1. Lift the right foot from the ground and balancing on your left leg bend forward at your waist. Lower the dumbbells as far as you can.
2. Reverse the movement and come back to the start position.
3. Repeat required number of times.
4. Switch the leg and repeat on the other side.

Fine Tips:

1. Try not to touch the off foot again and again on the ground.
2. You can bend the knee slightly if you feel comfortable.
3. Be extra careful while going down as overstretch can lead to hamstring pull.

Glutes Exercises

Weighted Bridge Lift

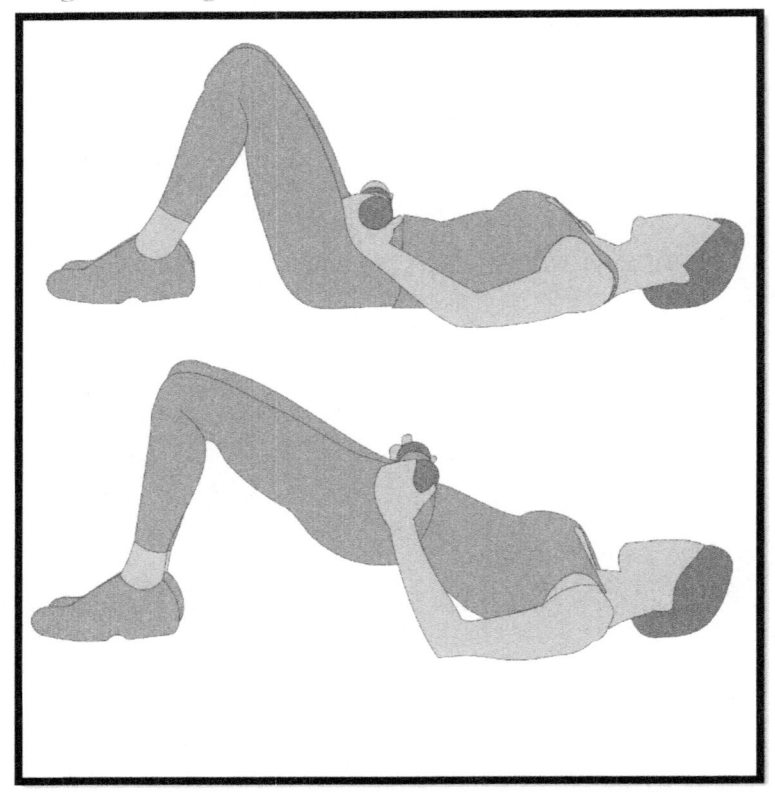

Strength Training with Dumbbells

Effect: This exercise mainly strengthens your gluteus muscles and to some extent lower back, abs, hip flexors and hamstring muscles.

Difficulty Level: Beginner

Start Position: Grab a dumbbell between your hands in front of the hip joint and lie down straight on your back with feet hip width apart. Bend your legs and place the feet flat on the floor about 1 feet away from the buttocks.

Steps:

1. Imprint your lower back (press it against the mat) squeeze your buttocks and raise the hips up, till your knees, hips and shoulders come in one line.
2. Pause at top position for 5 seconds and slowly lower the hips down to start position.
3. Repeat required number of times.

Fine Tips:

1. Keep your feet firmly grounded and do not let your knees flare out during the movement.
2. Keep breathing as you pause in the top position.

Calves Exercises

Standing Dumbbell Calf Raise

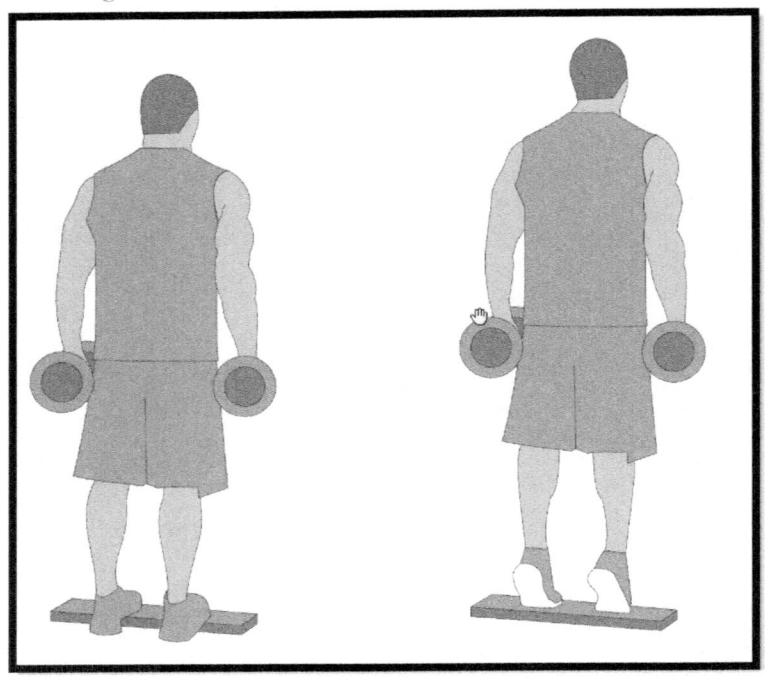

Strength Training with Dumbbells

Effect: This exercise helps to strengthen your calf muscles.

Difficulty Level: Intermediate

Start Position: Stand tall holding dumbbells by the side of your body with straight arms. Place the ball of your feet on a stable 2-3 inch high wooden bench so that your heel touches the floor.

Steps:

1. Raise the heels up contracting your calves.
2. Hold at the top position for a second and slowly lower the heels down to the start position.
3. Repeat required number of times.

Fine Tips:

1. Keep standing tall throughout the movement.

"I do some 400 m. repetition running for endurance on the court. I'll be in the gym lifting weights, or I'll be putting in a lot of core stability to work to improve my balance."

— Andy Murray

CHAPTER 6

Core Exercises

Dumbbell Side Plank Reach Rotate

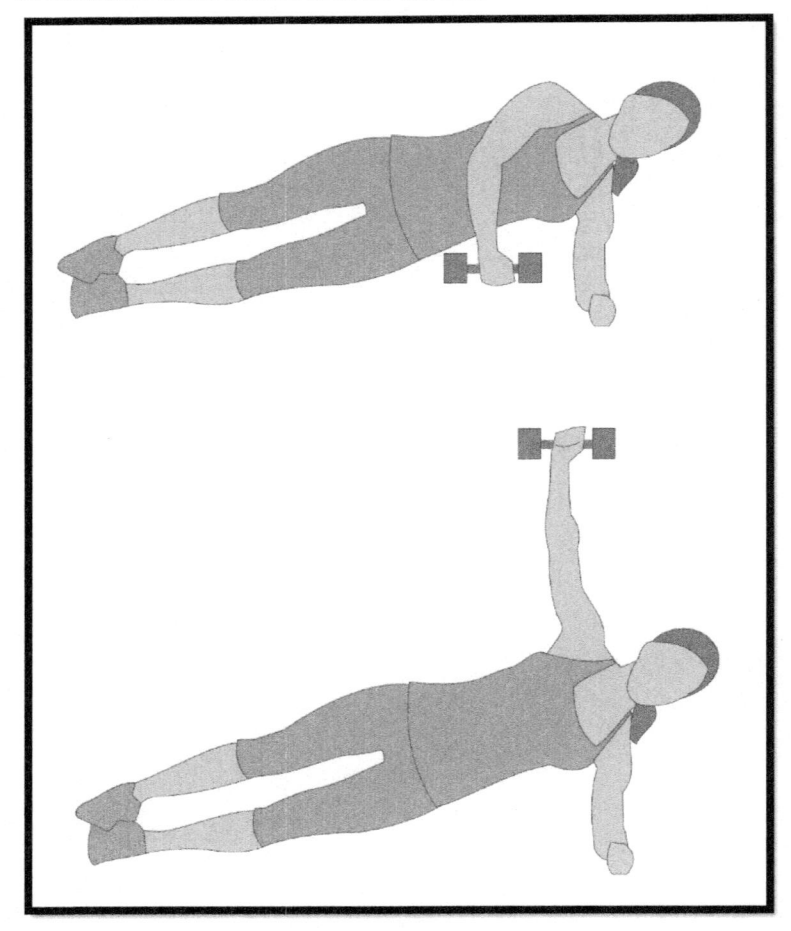

Strength Training with Dumbbells

Effect: This exercise mainly focuses on strengthening of obliques and to lesser degree on strengthening of gluteus, abs, lower back and shoulder muscles.

Difficulty Level: Intermediate

Start Position: Lie down on the left side of your body placing ankle over ankle. Next prop yourself up on left elbow and forearm and raise your hips up so that shoulder, hip and ankle come in one straight line. Grab a dumbbell in your right hand by the side of your body.

Steps:

1. Raise your right arm up so that it is perpendicular to the body.
2. Next reach under with your right hand till your chest becomes parallel to the floor.
3. Pause and twist back to starting position.
4. Repeat required number of times.

Fine Tips:

1. Brace your core throughout the movement.
2. Do not let your hips sag during the exercise.

Negative Sit-up

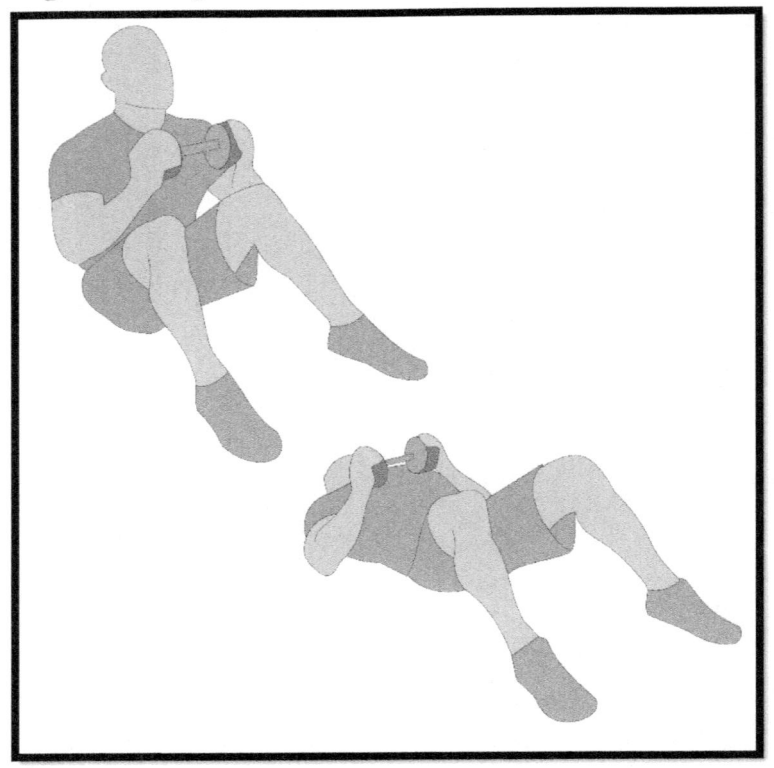

Strength Training with Dumbbells

Effect: Strengthening of lower abdominals and hip flexors

Difficulty Level: Intermediate

Start Position: Hold the dumbbell against your chest and sit in a sit up position with your knees bent at 90 degrees and feet flat on ground, hip width distance apart.

Steps:

1. Tuck in your abdomen and slowly lower your torso towards the floor. Breathe in.
2. Slowly return to the start position from the floor keeping your abdomen tucked in. Breathe out
3. Do required number of repetitions.

Fine Tips:

1. Keep your abdomen muscles engaged throughout the movement.
2. Movement should be slow and controlled.
3. Keep your head in line with your body throughout the movement.
4. Avoid curling your back as you come up from the floor.

Dumbbell Sit-ups

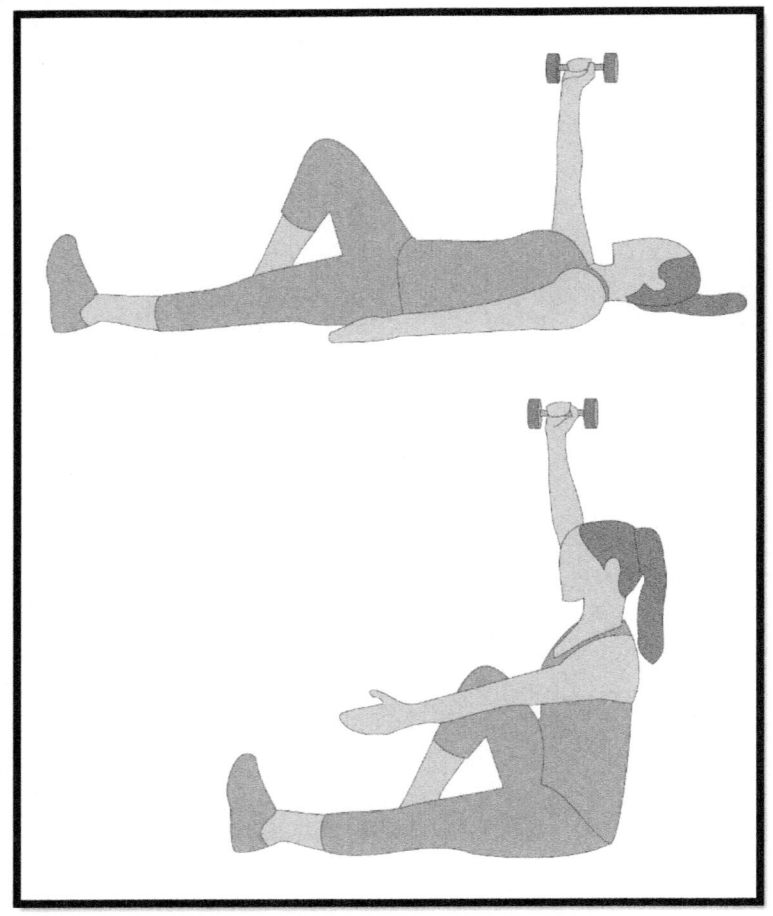

Strength Training with Dumbbells

Effect: This exercise helps to increase the strength and stability of core muscles along with the strengthening of supporting muscles that is hip flexors, hamstrings and glutes.

Difficulty Level: Intermediate

Start Position: Lie down straight with right leg bent and right foot on the floor. Grab a dumbbell in your right hand and hold it straight above the chest.

Steps:

1. Tuck in your abdomen and curl up to the sitting position keeping the dumbbell overhead.
2. Pause here and slowly return to the start position.
3. Repeat required number of times.
4. Repeat on the other side.

Fine Tips:

1. Keep your core engaged throughout the movement.
2. The movement should be slow and controlled.
3. Do the full range of movement with dumbbell overhead all the times.

Sit-ups with Dumbbells

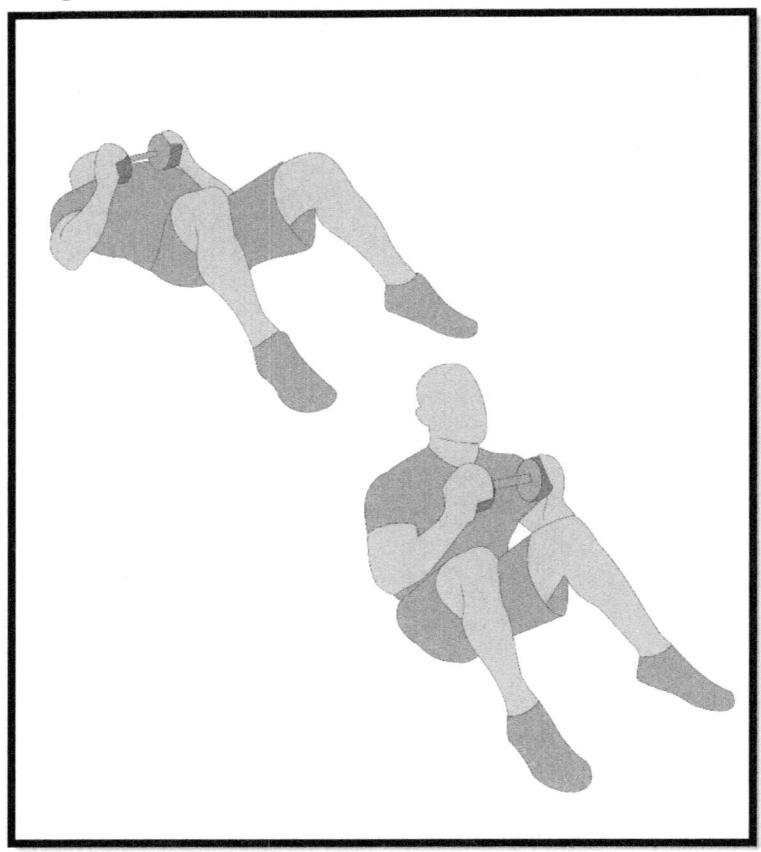

Strength Training with Dumbbells

Effect: This exercise increases the strength and stability of the core area by strengthening the lower back muscles, abdominals and hip flexors.

Difficulty Level: Intermediate

Start Position: Grab a dumbbell near your chest and lie down straight on your back with knees bent at 90 degrees and feet hip width apart, flat on the floor.

Steps:

1. Imprint your back (engage your core) and raise up till back of your forearm touches the thighs.
2. Pause here and then slowly return to the start position keeping your core engaged.
3. Repeat required number of times.

Fine Tips:

1. Keep your core engaged and the dumbbell close to your chest throughout the movement.
2. The movement should be slow and controlled without momentum helping in the movement.

"I've always overworked in the weight room. I love working with weights. I knew they'd give me the strength I needed."

— Florence Griffith Joyner

CHAPTER 7

Full Body Exercises

Dumbbell Raise with Jump

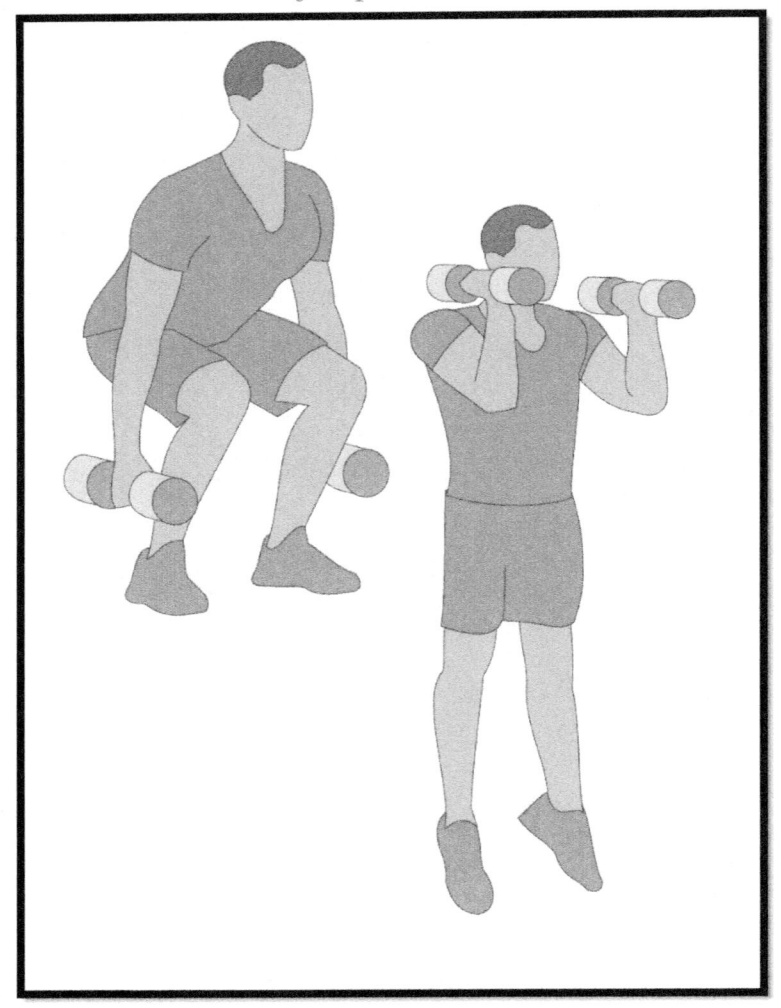

Strength Training with Dumbbells

Effect: This is a dynamic compound exercise focusing on shoulder, arms, lower back, core and legs strengthening.

Difficulty Level: Advanced

Start Position: Hold dumbbells in your hands with palms facing each other and arms by the side of your body, slightly flexed. Stand in partial squat position with abdomen tucked in, back tall and feet hip width distance apart.

Steps:

1. Take the dumbbells to the shoulder with a momentum and jump from partial squat position to stand tall position, pushing through the heel simultaneously.
2. Lower the dumbbells down and return to the start position.
3. Repeat required number of times.

Fine Tips:

1. Keep the dumbbells close to your body throughout the exercise.
2. Exercise should be performed in a quick manner.

Dumbbell One Arm Raise

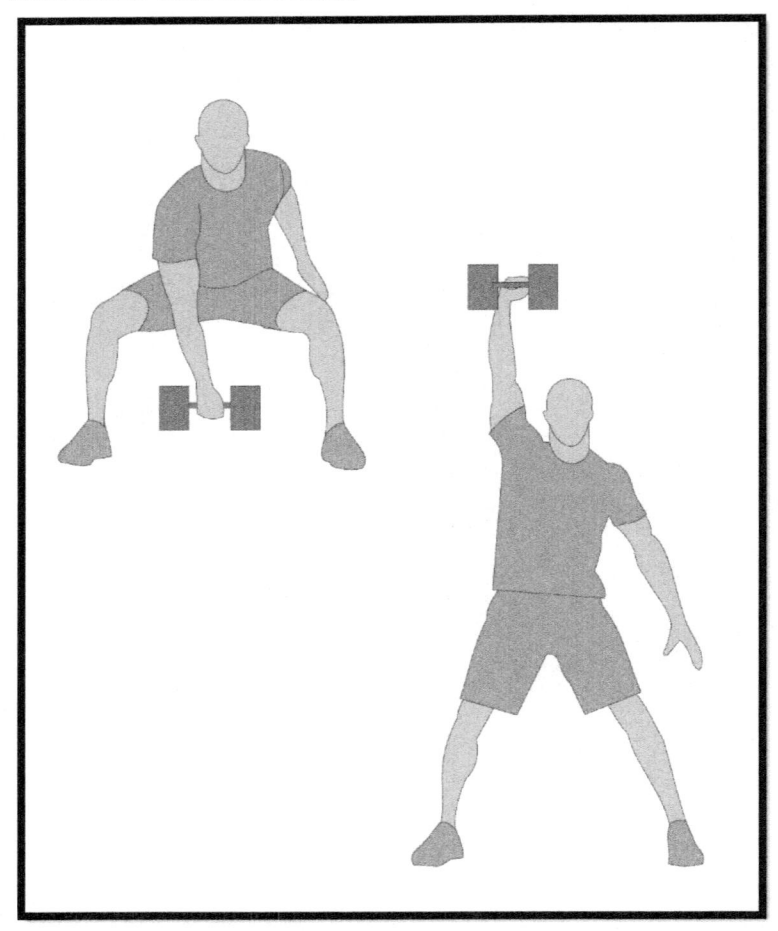

Strength Training with Dumbbells

Effect: This is a dynamic compound exercise focusing on strengthening of the arms and shoulders with core stability and lower body stability.

Difficulty Level: Advanced

Start Position: Grab dumbbell in one hand and stand tall with core engaged and feet more than hip width apart.

Steps:

1. Lower the dumbbell and bring it between the legs while bending at knees into half squat position.
2. In a quick manner push the dumbbell high up over the head and come to a stand tall position from the squat.
3. Repeat required number of times.

Fine Tips:

1. Keep the core engaged and neck tall throughout the exercise.
2. Use the momentum through the push from the leg to raise the dumbbell.

Dr. Monika Chopra's Fitness Sutra

Half Turkish Get-up Dumbbell Raise

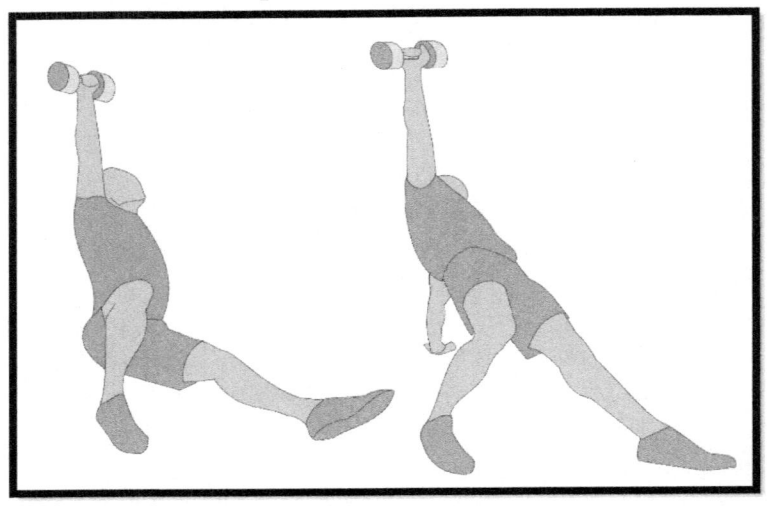

Strength Training with Dumbbells

Effect: It's a multiple joint movement focusing on full body strength and stability specifically targeting triceps, shoulders and hips.

Difficulty Level: Intermediate

Start Position: Sit upright with left leg straight in front and right leg bent with right foot flat on the floor. Place your left hand behind the left hip and hold dumbbell in your right hand with right arm extended up.

Steps:

1. Lift the hips into the air keeping the dumbbell raised towards the ceiling and your body weight supported on the left hand. Form a straight line from one hand to another and from shoulder to the leg.
2. Keep your core engaged and return to the start position.
3. Repeat required number of times and repeat on the other side.

Fine Tips:

1. Keep your core engaged throughout the movement.
2. Squeeze your glutes at the top of the movement while you pause there for a second.

Dr. Monika Chopra's Fitness Sutra

Dumbbell Chop

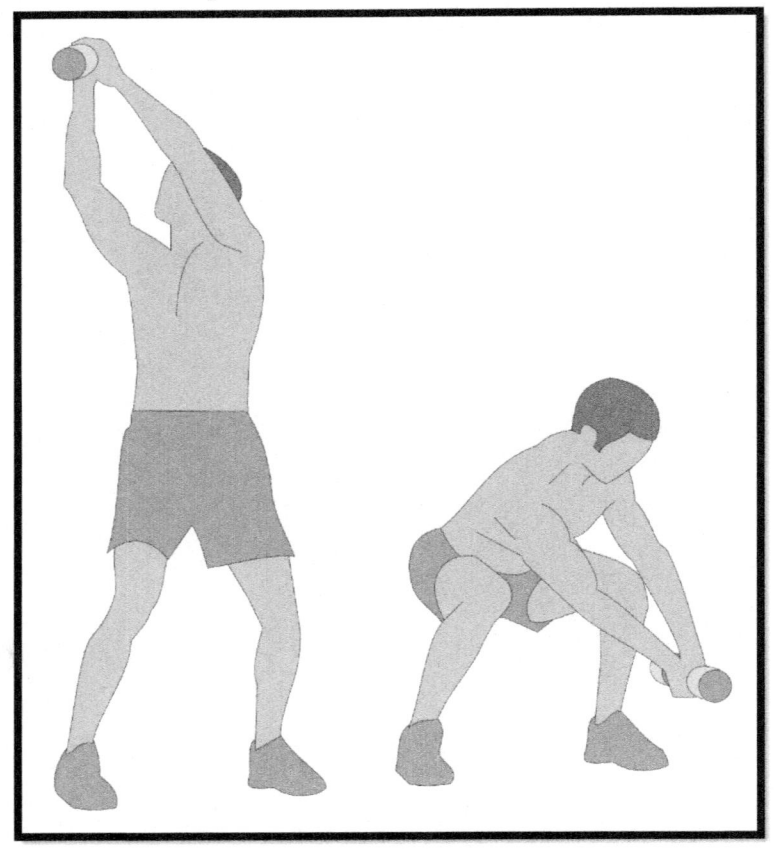

Strength Training with Dumbbells

Effect: This is a full body rotational exercise focusing on strengthening of lower abdominals and obliques. It improves the rotational movement through lower back and hips.

Difficulty Level: Beginner

Start Position: Grab the dumbbell with both hands above right shoulder standing with knees slightly flexed.

Steps:

1. With a rotational movement at the trunk, take the dumbbell towards the left hip, straightening the arms.
2. Repeat required number of times.
3. Repeat on the other side.

Fine Tips:

1. The rotational movement should happen from hip and core and not from shoulder.
2. Avoid hyperextending of back and keep it neutral throughout the movement.

Single Arm Dumbbell Snatch

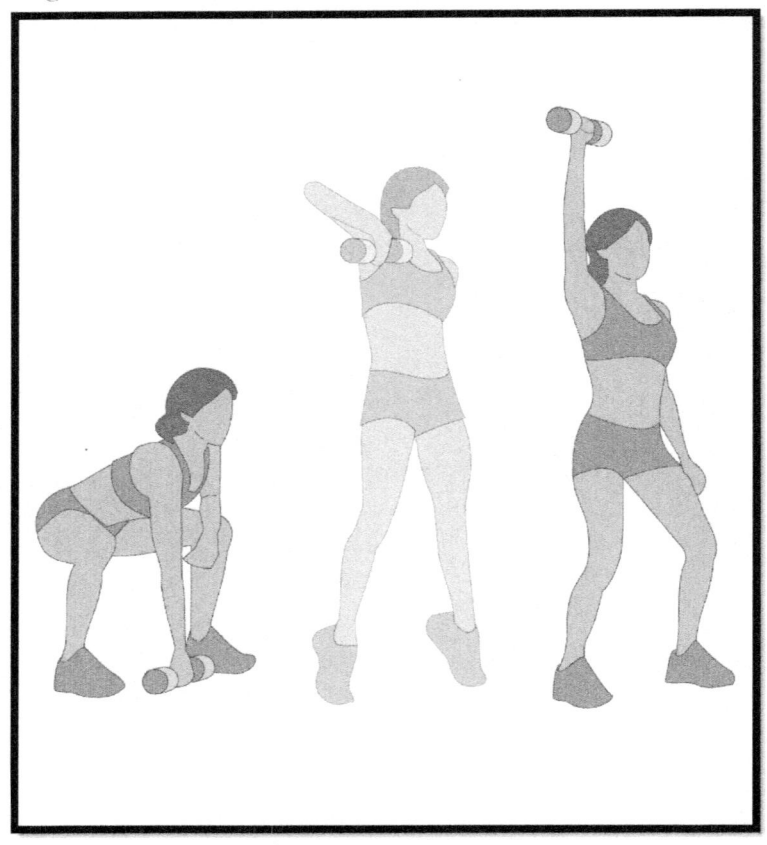

Strength Training with Dumbbells

Effect: This is a full body coordination and strengthening exercise focusing mainly on strengthening of arms, shoulders and upper back.

Difficulty Level: Advanced

Start Position: Grab the dumbbell using overhand grip, other arm by the side of your body and stand in a partial squat position with feet little apart than the shoulders.

Steps:

1. Descend your hips towards the floor till your knees bend at 90 degrees holding the dumbbell down in front of your body.
2. From the dumbbell in the down position raise the dumbbell and push it towards the ceiling overhead straightening the legs. Raise your body on the balls of the feet.
3. As the dumbbell reaches the highest point bend the elbow and get the weight down to the shoulder with the palm facing forward.
4. Return to the start position.
5. Repeat required number of times.
6. Repeat on the other side.

Fine Tips:

1. Always keep dumbbell close to your body.
2. Keep your core engaged throughout the movement.
3. The movement should start from hips and glutes.

Overhead Dumbbell Squat

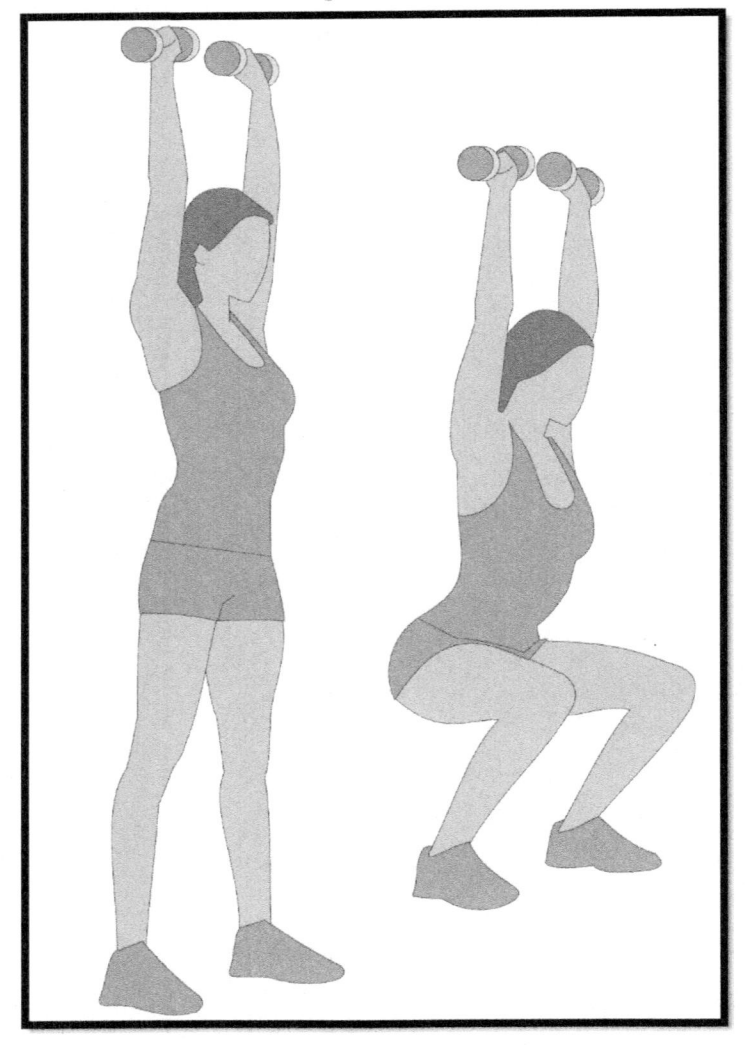

Strength Training with Dumbbells

Effect: This is a multiple joint exercise focusing on strengthening of lower body and arms along with increasing core stability.

Difficulty Level: Intermediate

Start Position: Grab the dumbbells overhead with arms little wider than shoulder width and palms facing forward. Stand tall with feet little wider than shoulder width and toes pointing outwards.

Steps:

1. From the start position lower into the squat position pulling the tail bone (hips) down towards the ground till the thighs come parallel to the floor.
2. Pause in this position and raise back to the start position.
3. Repeat required number of times.

Fine Tips:

1. The elbows should remain straight overhead throughout the movement.
2. The knees should not cave in as you lower down into squat position.
3. Keep your back tall and core engaged throughout the movement.

Dr. Monika Chopra's Fitness Sutra

Dumbbell Split Jump

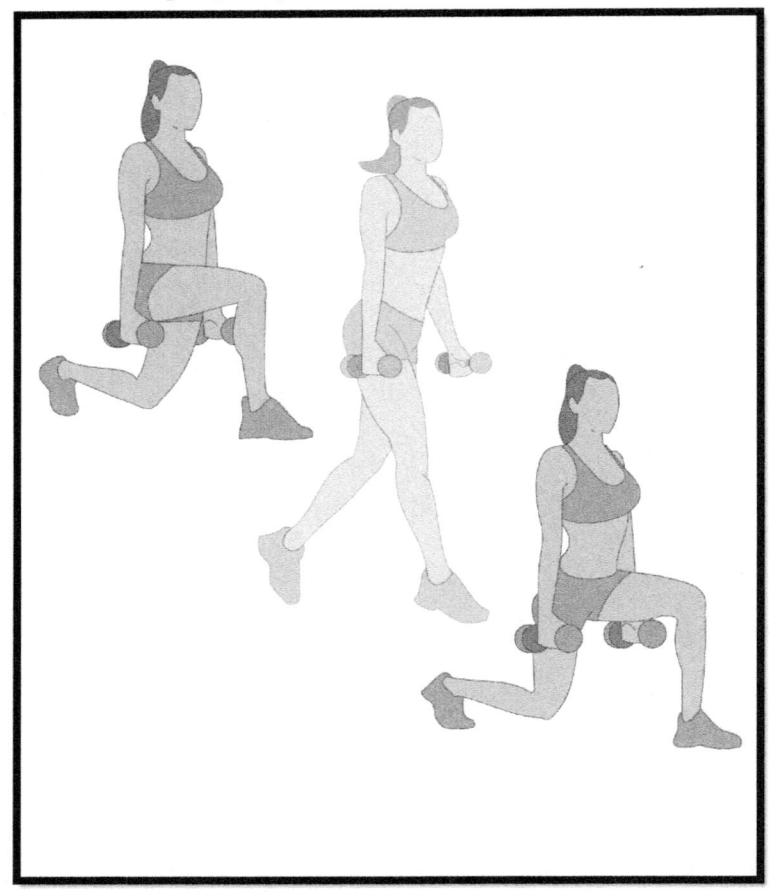

Strength Training with Dumbbells

Effect: This exercise increases the endurance of whole body working on the jumping power and strength of the legs.

Difficulty Level: Advanced

Start Position: Grab dumbbells in your hands with arms straight, by the side of your body and palms facing each other. Stand tall with feet hip width apart.

Steps:

1. Take your left leg behind lowering the left knee towards the ground in a lunge keeping the right shin vertical to the floor.
2. Pushing through both the feet, jump and switch the legs in the air landing softly in the lunge position with opposite leg forward.
3. Immediately repeat the movement switching the leg.
4. Repeat required number of times.

Fine Tips:

1. The jump should be as high as possible to get the best results.
2. The movement should be derived from front foot heel.
3. Keep your torso tall throughout the movement.

Dumbbell Reverse Lunge High Knee and Press

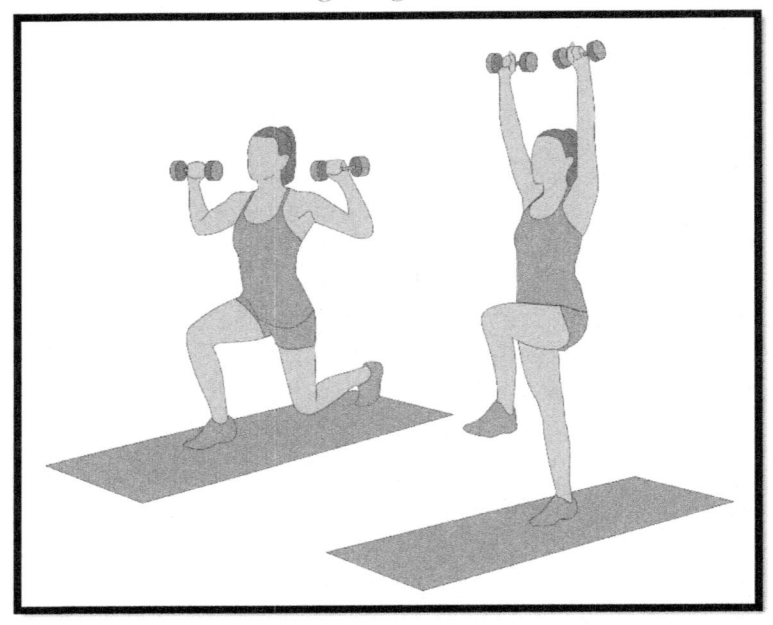

Strength Training with Dumbbells

Effect: This exercise increases the endurance of your body with simultaneously increasing the strength of your legs and arms. It also increases the mobility and flexibility of legs and hips.

Difficulty Level: Advanced

Start Position: Grab the dumbbells in your hands at the shoulder level. Take a large step behind taking your left foot behind, lowering the left knee towards the ground; keeping the right shin vertical to the ground.

Steps:

1. Pushing through your right foot take your left foot forward and raise your left knee towards the chest simultaneously pressing the dumbbells overhead.
2. Reverse the movement and return to the start position. Repeat required number of times.
3. Repeat on the other side.

Fine Tips:

1. Keep your torso tall and core engaged throughout the movement.

Dr. Monika Chopra's Fitness Sutra

Dumbbell Full Squat Press

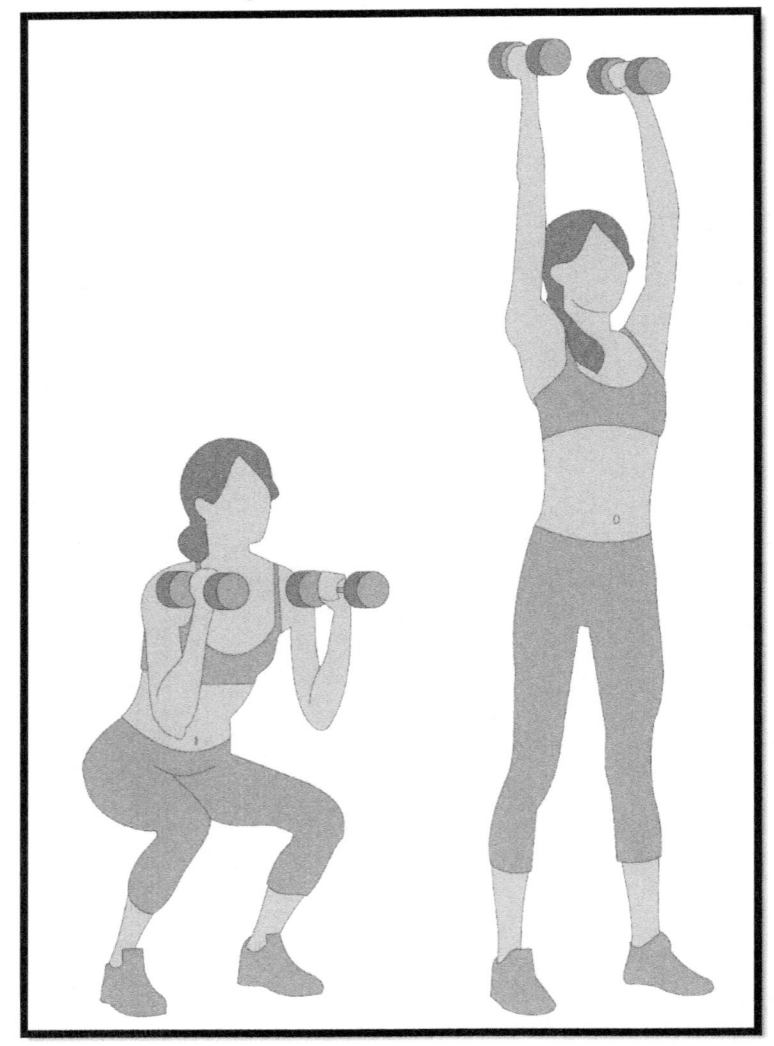

Strength Training with Dumbbells

Effect: This exercise helps to strengthen shoulder front muscles. Arm back muscles, hip and thigh muscles and total body power and explosiveness.

Difficulty Level: Advanced

Start Position: Stand tall with feet hip width distance apart. Grab dumbbells in your hands with palms facing in and rest them at shoulder level.

Steps:

1. Come to a full squat position with your thighs parallel to floor and dumbbells at the shoulder level.
2. In an explosive movement with as much force as you can come to the standing position pushing the dumbbells overhead, extending the arms straight and palms still facing in.
3. Return to the start position.
4. Repeat required number of times.

Fine Tips:

1. Keep your back tall and core engaged throughout the movement.
2. Go as low in squat as you comfortably can.

Dr. Monika Chopra's Fitness Sutra

Jumping Jacks with Dumbbells

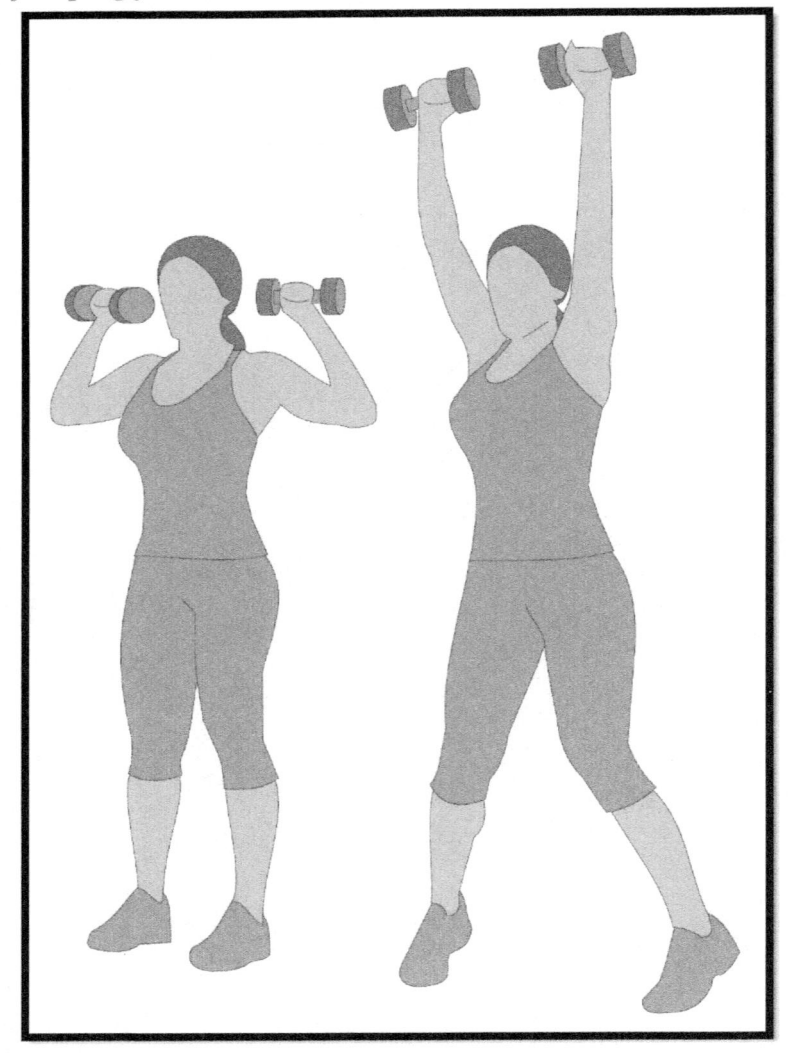

Strength Training with Dumbbells

Effect: This exercise focuses mainly on strengthening of arms and shoulder muscles.

Difficulty Level: Beginner

Start Position: Grab dumbbells in your hands with palms facing forward, elbows bent and at shoulder level. Stand tall with feet shoulder width apart.

Steps:

1. Push the dumbbells overhead as you jump and move the feet apart.
2. Reverse the movement and return to start position.
3. Repeat required number of times.

Dumbbell Windmill

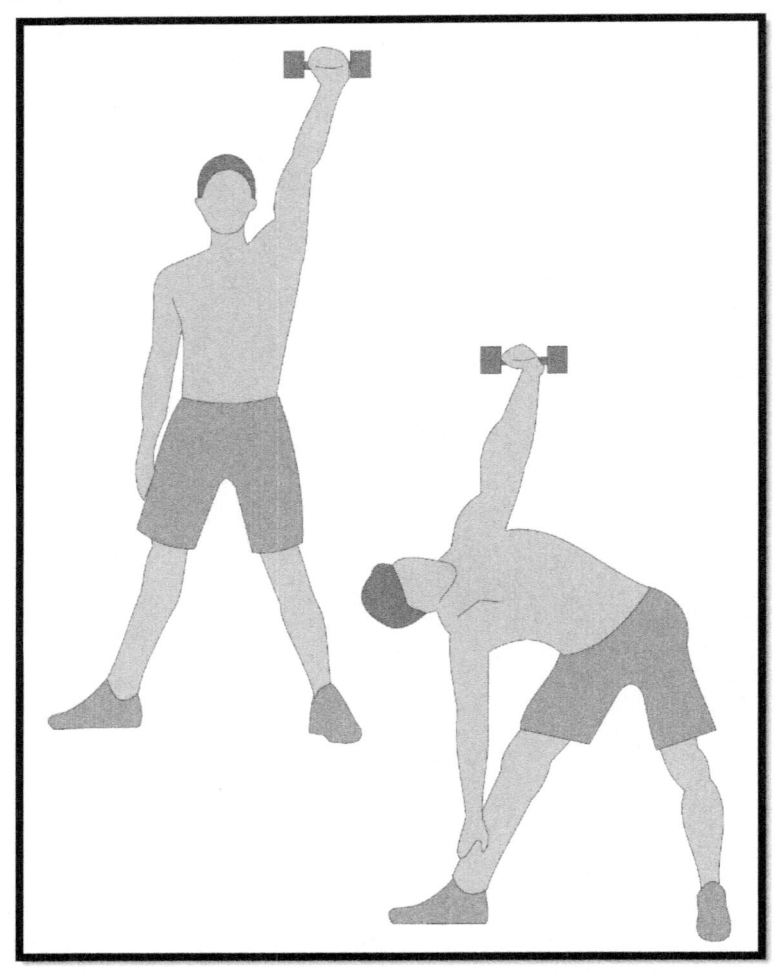

Strength Training with Dumbbells

Effect: This exercise helps to increase shoulder muscles strength and stability and improves core strength.

Difficulty Level: Intermediate

Start Position: Grab dumbbell in left hand, palm facing forward and push it overhead standing tall with feet shoulder width apart.

Steps:

1. Start the movement by hitching left hip to left side and bending down, rotating your core trying to reach your right foot with right hand. Keep your left hand with dumbbell pushed overhead.
2. Look upwards towards the dumbbell keeping your arm and core rotated.
3. Reverse the movement and return to the start position.
4. Switch hands and repeat on left side.
5. Repeat required number of times.

Fine Tips:

1. The movement should be slow and controlled.

CHAPTER 8

Cool-Down Exercises

Strength Training with Dumbbells

Cool down exercises should always be performed after intensive workout to bring the body back to its normal state. Full body stretches are good cool down exercises. The body is in a very compliant state after exercises. Thus the stretches performed at this time also help to increase the flexibility of the body.

Cool down stretch guidelines
1. Move into the stretched position (where you can feel slight tension) slowly.
2. Inhale and exhale deeply and slowly and let the stretching muscle relax.
3. Hold the stretch for 15 seconds and then slowly return to start position.
4. Perform each stretch twice.

Some stretches which are very beneficial for the body are as follows:

Upper Body Stretch
1. <u>Triceps Stretch (Forward Arm Stretch):</u>

Major muscles worked - rhomboids, deltoids and triceps brachii. Stand tall with your shoulders levelled and facing forwards and feet hip width distance apart. Extend your right arm to the side at shoulder level with palm facing forward. Move the arm forward and take it across the chest as if to wrap your chest with your arm. Bring the right hand around your left shoulder blade walking your fingertips towards your upper spine to the extent it is comfortable.

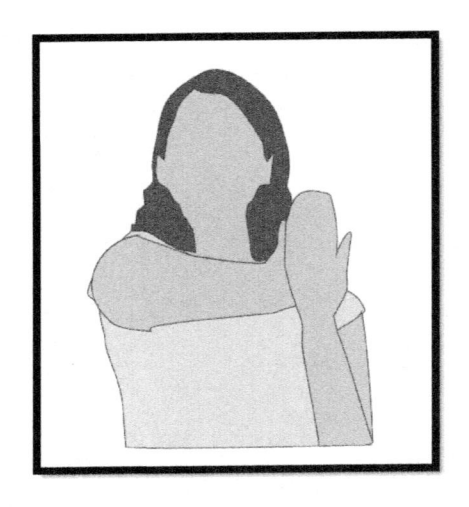

Feel the stretch on the outside of your right arm, right shoulder and upper back. Breathe deeply into the thoracic spine and upper back, trying to release the stretching muscles. To increase the stretch you may give a slight push at the elbow of the wrapped arm, pulling it towards your chest. Relax. Repeat the above procedure for the left side.

2. <u>Pectoral Stretch (Backward Arm Stretch)</u>:

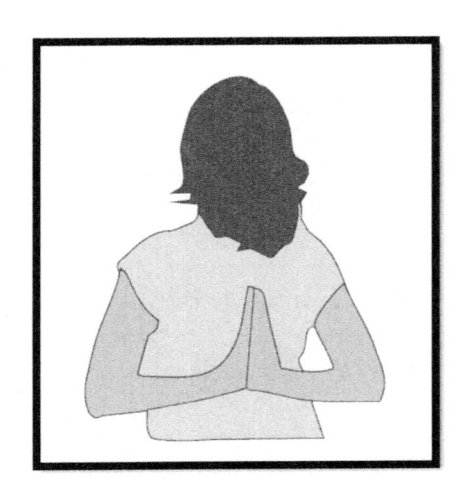

Major muscles worked - pectoralis major and deltoids. Stand tall with your shoulders levelled and facing forward and feet hip width distance apart. Extend your arms to the sides making a "T". Bend your arms at the elbows and bring both hands behind your back till the tip of middle fingers touch each other with little fingers of both hands pressing against the back. Start pushing the middle fingers up slowly. Try to bring all the fingers of left hand in contact with fingers of right hand. Slide the fingers up the spine till the stretch is comfortable. Inhale deeply while stretching the muscles of shoulder, chest, arms and fingers, relaxing them.

3. <u>Latissimus Dorsi And Triceps Stretch (Upward Arm Stretch)</u>:

Major muscles worked - Latissimus dorsi and Triceps brachii
Extend your right arm to the side with palm facing up. Raise the arm towards the ceiling and then bend at the elbow till your fingertips reach the spine between your shoulder blades. Walk your fingertips down the spine. Feel the stretch on the outer side of your right arm, upper back and the right side of your trunk. Hold this position and breathe deeply trying to release the stretching muscles of the upper back and around the spine. Come to the start position. Repeat the above procedure for the left side.

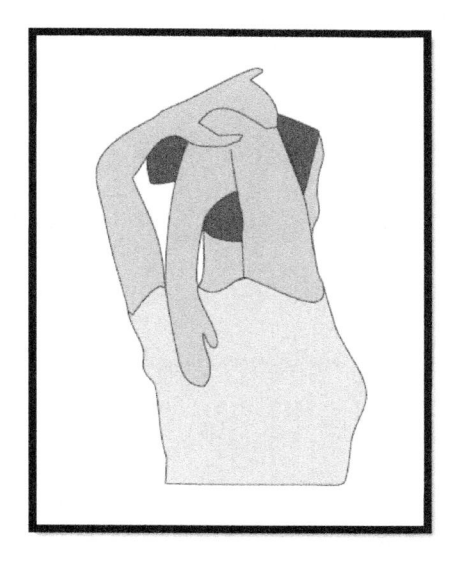

Lower Body Stretch

1. Figure Of Four Forward Bend:

Major muscles worked - gluteus maximus and erector spinae.

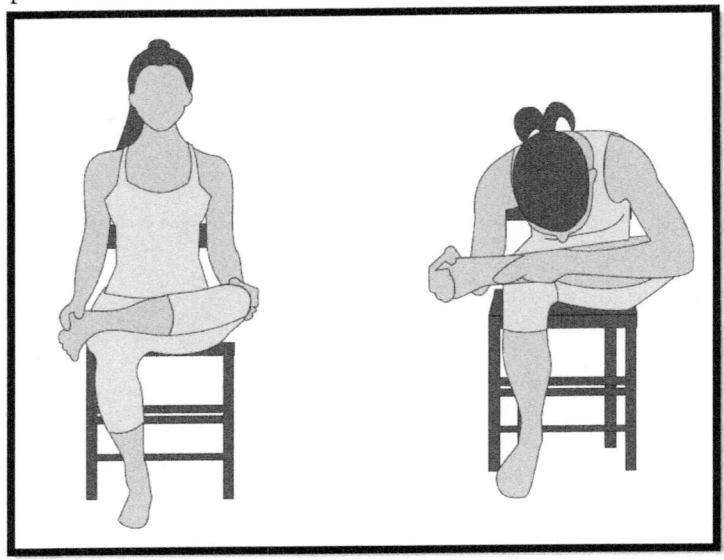

Sit tall with feet firmly placed on the ground, hip width distance apart. Place your left ankle over the right knee making a figure of 4 with the legs. Stretch your spine in this position trying to free your hip joint. Let the knee go down under the effect of gravity, opening the left hip joint. Bend forward from this position, leading with your chest while still looking ahead. Breathe while stretching and release the spine and hip joint slowly. Drop your body down towards the floor. Feel the increase in stretch in the hip and spine region. Hold this position. To come out of

Strength Training with Dumbbells

the above position, raise your spine up, keeping it straight while still keeping the neck and shoulders relaxed. Keep pushing through the right foot into the ground to maintain balance. As the spine comes in an upright position, raise the head and look in front. Come to the start position. Repeat on the other side.

2. <u>Thigh Stretch (Quadriceps Stretch)</u>:

Stand tall with your abdomen tucked in and feet hip width distance apart. Hold a wall or stationary object for balance, Grasp your left foot with your left hand and pull so that your left heel moves towards your left buttock (maintain proper alignment to avoid stress on your knee). You should feel the stretch along the front of your left thigh. Repeat on the other leg.

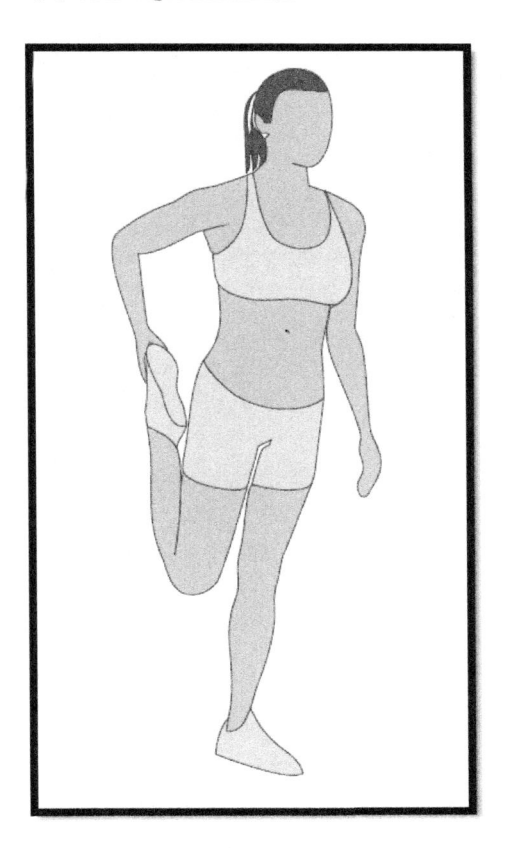

3. <u>Hamstring Stretch:</u>

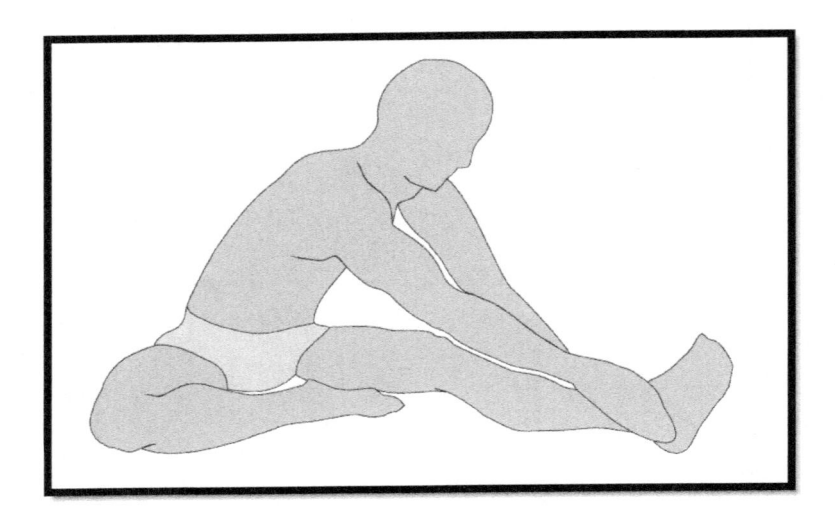

Major muscles worked - Hamstrings and erector spinae. Sit tall in a long sitting position on the floor with your legs hip width distance apart and stretched in front of you. Bend your right leg and place the sole of right foot against the inner side of left thigh, above the knee. Keep your shoulders and hips squared (facing forward). Bend forward at your hips (keeping your back straight and leading with the heart) and move your torso towards your left knee. Be sure to keep your left leg in neutral position with your left toes pointing up. Feel the stretch in your back and hamstring muscles. Switch the leg and repeat on the other side keeping your right leg stretched in front of you.

4. <u>Calf Muscle Stretch:</u>

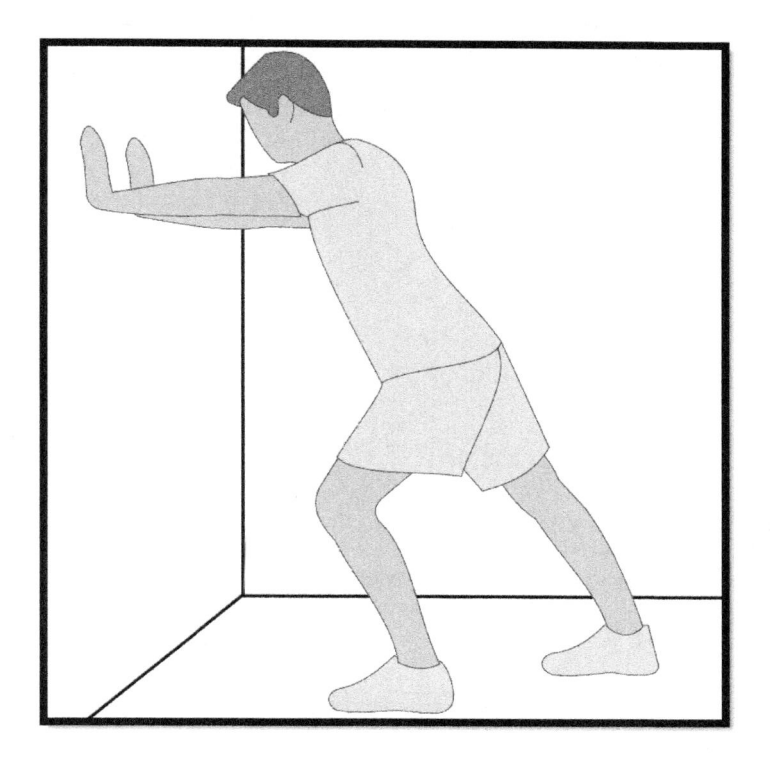

Major muscles involved: Soleus and gastrocnemius.
Stand with your right foot flat on the floor about 1 foot away from the wall (right leg bent) and the left leg stretched straight behind with left heel touching the floor. Place your hands on the wall and bend forwards, keeping your back straight. Feel the stretch behind your left leg. Repeat on the other side.

CHAPTER 9

Importance of Diet

Importance of proper diet in your journey to strength & fitness cannot be overstated. This chapter will give you simple tips on what to eat as balanced diet to maintain a lean but strong physique.

1. Eat protein with each meal – adequate amount of protein consumption is essential for muscle tissue recovery during strength training program. Whole proteins should be part of each of your meals. Proteins keep you full for longer time thus helping in fat loss. Protein rich foods have a higher thermic effect, thus more of the meal is burned during digestion. Each day, one should eat 1g of protein for every 1 pound of body weight.

2. Eat vegetables with each meal – vegetables are fibre rich and thus fill you up with less carbs intake. Fibre also improves digestion. Vegetables contain many valuable vitamins, phytochemicals, and antioxidants for better health. You should aim to eat at least half a plate of veggies at each meal. Vegetables contain lots of fibre that would help in your bowel movements that may otherwise get adversely affected with a high protein diet.

3. Limit your carbohydrate intake – carbohydrates are high calorie food. If you are doing strength training to reduce body fat you should limit your carbohydrate intake thus limiting calorie intake.

4. Avoid processed food – avoid processed food and try to consume food mostly in natural state. Processed foods (generally all the eatables that are

made in factories like soda, cookies, cereals (including bars), frozen food etc.) are invariably high in sugar & salt. Sugar can be disguised as other ingredients like HFCS (i.e. High Fructose Corn Syrup). Factories put in high amounts of sugar & fats to compensate for the loss of taste that invariably occurs due to mass production & packaging.

5. <u>Eat good fats</u> – fat do not necessarily make you fat. Considerate amount of fat is actually required while strength training. Fat keeps you full for longer periods of time and provide essential fatty acids. Include some nuts & dry fruits in your meal plan for snack times.

6. <u>Drink lots of water</u> – It is essential to keep yourself hydrated all the time; especially during workouts as you tend to lose a lot of water through sweating. Dehydration from lack of drinking may cause headaches for some folks. Also you need water for proper muscle recovery. Do not go by any thumb rules for water intake - just ensure to drink as & when you feel thirsty. If you do not feel the need to empty your bladder every few hours, then it's a sign that you are not taking in enough water to flush all the toxins.

CHAPTER 10

Training Regimes

Dr. Monika Chopra's Fitness Sutra

Beginners' Regime

In 1st week, do 2 sets of 8 repetitions each.
In 2nd week, do 2 sets of 10 repetitions each.
In the 3rd week, do 2 sets of 12 repetitions each.

Day 1 & Day 5

Lower body
- Dumbbell Step
- Goblet Squat with Pulses
- Curtsy Lunge
- Romanian Deadlift
- Weighted Bridge Lift
- Standing Dumbbell Calf Raise

Core
- Negative Sit-up

Full body
- Dumbbell Chop
- Overhead Dumbbell Squat
- Jumping Jacks with Dumbbells

Strength Training with Dumbbells

Day 3 & Day 7

Upper body
- Hammer-Curl
- Reverse Biceps Curl
- Seated Dumbbell Triceps Extension
- Overhead Dumbbell Press
- Seated Overhead Dumbbell Press
- Dumbbell Front Raise
- Dumbbell Shoulder Shrug
- Seated Dumbbell Palm-up Wrist Curl
- Dumbbell Bench Press
- Flat Dumbbell Crush Press
- 3-point Support Dumbbell Row
- Bent-over Dumbbell Sideways Raise

Core
- Sit-ups with Dumbbells

Full Body
- Dumbbell Chop
- Jumping Jacks with Dumbbells

Dr. Monika Chopra's Fitness Sutra

Intermediates' Regime

In 1st week, do 2 sets of 10 repetitions each.
In 2nd week, do 3 sets of 8 repetitions each.
In the 3rd week, do 3 sets of 10 repetitions each.

Day 1 & Day 5

Lower Body
- Dumbbell Diagonal Lunge
- Walking Dumbbell Lunge
- Goblet Squat with Pulses
- Bulgarian Split Lunge
- Single Leg Dumbbell Deadlift

Core
- Sit-ups with Dumbbells

Full Body
- Half Turkish Get-up Dumbbell Raise
- Single Arm Dumbbell Snatch
- Dumbbell Split Jump
- Dumbbell Reverse Lunge High Knee and Press

Strength Training with Dumbbells

Day 3 & Day 7

Upper Body
- Reverse Biceps Curl
- Bent-over Triceps Kickback
- Seated Side Lateral Raise
- Dumbbell L-Arm Lateral Raise
- Overhead Dumbbell Press
- Dumbbell Pull Over the Head
- Seated Dumbbell Palm-up Wrist Curl
- Flat Dumbbell Crush Press
- Incline Dumbbell Chest Fly
- Supported Incline Chest Dumbbell Row
- 3-point Support Dumbbell Row

Core
- Dumbbell Sit-ups
- Negative Sit-up

Full Body
- Overhead Dumbbell Squat
- Dumbbell Windmill

Advanced Regime

In 1st week, do 3 sets of 10 repetitions each.
In 2nd week, do 3 sets of 12 repetitions each.
In the 3rd week, do 3 sets of 12 repetitions each.

Day 1 & Day 5

Lower Body
- Dumbbell Lunge and Rotation
- Side Lunge Jump off
- Goblet Squat with Pulses
- Bulgarian Split Lunge
- Romanian Deadlift

Core
- Dumbbell Sit-ups

Full Body
- Dumbbell Raise with Jump
- Single Arm Dumbbell Snatch
- Dumbbell Split Jump
- Dumbbell Windmill

Strength Training with Dumbbells

Day 3 & Day 7

Upper Body
- Split Stance Dumbbell Curl
- Bent-over Triceps Kickback
- Alternate Dumbbell Incline Bench Press
- Side Lying Lateral Raise
- Upright Row
- Dumbbell Swing
- Seated Dumbbell Palm-up Wrist Curl
- Dumbbell "T" Push-Ups
- Dumbbell Rowing
- Renegade Row
- Bent-over Dumbbell Sideways Raise

Core
- Dumbbell Side Plank Reach Rotate

Full Body
- Dumbbell Raise with Jump
- Dumbbell One Arm Raise
- Dumbbell Full Squat Press

Bonus

I hope you liked the book and have already started doing these exercises. Please give me a review on Amazon

https://www.fitness-sutra.com/go?id=131276

I have created easy to use quick reference charts of the regimes (beginners / intermediate / advanced) suggested in the previous chapter of this book. These can be downloaded as ready printable files from

https://www.fitness-sutra.com/go?id=131128

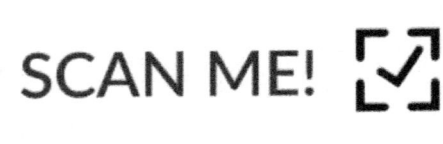

You can also subscribe to my mailing list to get more tips & motivation to do these exercises.

Strength Training with Dumbbells

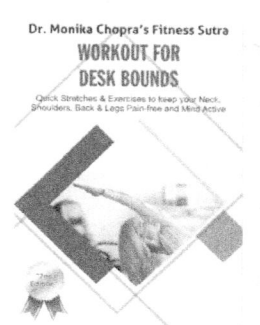

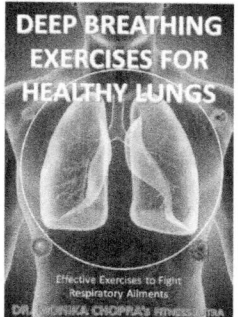

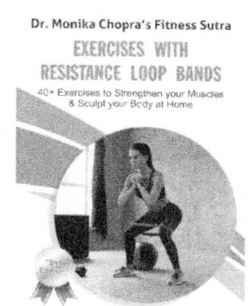

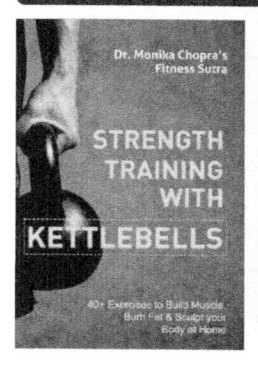

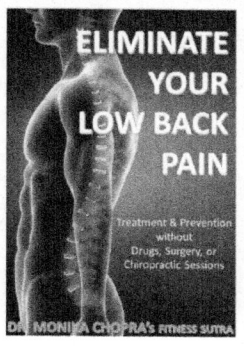

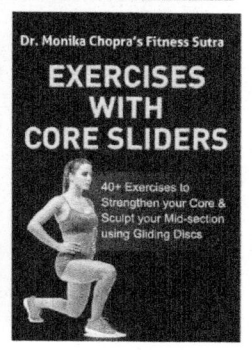

https://www.fitness-sutra.com/go?id= 132576

Printed in Great Britain
by Amazon